Introduction to

Electromyography and
Nerve Conduction Testing

Second Edition

D1546710

Introduction to

Electromyography and
Nerve Conduction Testing

Second Edition

Laboratory Exercises Included

John L. Echternach, EdD, PT, ECS, FAPTA
School of Physical Therapy
Old Dominion University
Norfolk, Virginia

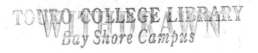
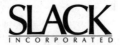
SLACK
INCORPORATED

An innovative information, education and management company
6900 Grove Road • Thorofare, NJ 08086

BS

Library of Congress Cataloging-in-Publication Data

Echternach, John L.
   Introduction to electromyography and nerve conduction testing / John
L. Echternach.-- 2nd ed.
      p. ; cm.
Includes bibliographical references and index.
   ISBN 1-55642-529-5 (pbk. : alk. paper)
   1. Electromyography--Handbooks, manuals, etc. 2. Neural
conduction--Testing--Handbooks, manuals, etc. 3. Physical therapists.
   [DNLM: 1. Neural Conduction--Laboratory Manuals. 2.
Electromyography--Laboratory Manuals. WL 25 E18i 2002] I. Title.
   RC77.5 .E24 2002
   616.7'407547--dc21

                                                                    2002010364

Printed in the United States of America.

Published by: SLACK Incorporated
                     6900 Grove Road
                     Thorofare, NJ 08086 USA
                     Telephone: 856-848-1000
                     Fax: 856-853-5991
                     www.slackbooks.com

   Last digit is print number: 10   9   8   7   6   5   4   3   2   1

10/21/03

Dedication

To the individuals who taught nerve conduction velocity and electromyography for the American Physical Therapy Association (APTA) Professional Enhancement Program (PEP) in the 1970s.

Secondly, to the individuals who have been certified by the American Board of Physical Therapy Specialists as Electrophysiologic Certified Specialist (ECS). I would like to acknowledge the small group of individuals who practice in this area who are always willing to do the extra work and who expend an enormous amount of energy to advance this area of practice among physical therapists.

Finally, to my wife Jeanne, who has fully supported me in my professional life.

Contents

Acknowledgments

In addition to the clinicians mentioned in the Preface, I would like to thank my colleagues at Old Dominion University in the School of Physical Therapy for their support in developing this text, as well as thank Debbie Miller and Don Emminger, graphic designers, Academic Technology Services, for the illustrations in the text. I would also like to acknowledge the great help and patience shown by Carrie N. Kotlar in the process of developing this second edition. In addition, I would like to thank my wife, Jeanne, for her continuing patience and support as I have devoted time to my professional interests, always with her encouragement and assistance.

About the Author

John (Jack) Echternach has been a physical therapist for more than 45 years. He graduated from West Chester University, West Chester, Pa, with a bachelor of science degree in health and physical education. Following this, he attended the University of Pennsylvania and obtained a certificate in physical therapy. Shortly after graduation, Dr. Echternach was commissioned as a physical therapy officer in the US Public Health Service where he served for the next 24 years. During this time, Dr. Echternach served many positions, from staff physical therapist to chief of the physical therapy department to the officer-in-charge of occupational and physical therapy activities in the Division of Hospitals and Clinics of the US Health Service. During his career in the US Public Health Service, Dr. Echternach obtained a master's degree in anatomy from the University of Maryland and a doctor of education in higher education/administration from the College of William and Mary, Williamsburg, Va.

Following his career in the US Public Health Service, Dr. Echternach became a faculty member at Old Dominion University, where he began the Physical Therapy Education Program and remained its director until 1992. During his time at Old Dominion University, he has also served as chairman of the School of the Community Health Professions and Physical Therapy. Dr. Echternach continues his career as a faculty member at Old Dominion University with the designation of professor and eminent scholar in the School of Physical Therapy.

Dr. Echternach remains active in conducting an electrophysiological testing practice working with primarily upper extremity problems. Dr. Echternach has published several professional papers on a variety of topics and authored chapters in several textbooks. He has served as editor of two textbooks and has authored two books relating to physical therapy practice.

Preface

The idea for a beginners' text and laboratory manual in electromyography and nerve conduction studies grew out of my early experiences in teaching electromyography and nerve conduction studies in the early 1970s. Initially, I was invited to present information about nerve conduction velocity (NCV) testing and electromyography (EMG) at state chapter meetings and an occasional university workshop where I would be a part of a group of speakers. In one instance, I was the only speaker for a 3-day workshop. During these early experiences, I would often prepare hand-out materials to help those attending the workshop learn techniques in laboratory sessions.

Later, I was asked to join a remarkable group of clinicians, who were sponsored to give 5-day workshops on these topics for the Professional Enhancement Program of the American Physical Therapy Association. The physical therapists who were part of this venture were Cathy Robertson, who coordinated these workshops; Art Nelson; Roger Nelson; Alan Stone; Austin Summer, MD; and also Arnold Tripp. The physical therapists in the group were doing electromyography and nerve conduction studies at a time when very few other members of the profession were involved, and our primary purpose in these workshops was to offer information on helping people get started doing NCV and EMG examinations. As this group worked together, materials were developed and handed out at workshops, and some of these materials resemble the materials that are in this beginners' manual.

In the middle 1970s, as a practicing clinician in the US Public Health Service, I was doing electromyography and nerve conduction studies, which were routine clinical activities of the physical therapy staff. The staff with whom I was practicing as a clinician was frequently asked to provide training for physical therapists and physical therapy students on clinical affiliations. Clinicians would come and spend 1 to 2 weeks with us to learn as much as possible about EMG and nerve conduction studies. During this time I and another member of my staff, Roy R. Taylor, who has subsequently become a physician, wrote the first version of this beginners' manual.

Over the years, I have rewritten much of the material, and I have continued to use it in workshops such as those I have taught in Kansas City in association with Paul Giesenhagan. I have found that having such a format for teaching workshops was extremely helpful. I also found that as I began teaching nerve conduction studies and electromyography to entry-level physical therapy students, I was able to use a similar format (a beginners' text with laboratory exercises) for this teaching environment.

Because I have used this workbook approach in the classroom and in workshops now for many years, I felt it was time to see if this material could be useful to a wider audience. The intended use of this beginners' text is that it always be supplemented by the use of other texts and materials. The bibliography includes a variety of sources that could be used in conjunction with this text. While the beginners' text and laboratory exercises could stand alone in some areas, they would best be supplemented by additional readings and the use of additional materials. Two suggestions are offered: one is that basic texts be used and the other is that a videotape or CD of abnormal electromyography potentials be used for one laboratory session. If this text is used in conjunction with the other materials, as I have suggested, I feel that it can prepare an individual to do clinical testing, both nerve conduction studies and EMG, under the supervision of an experienced examiner.

In a text such as this, very few of the ideas offered are original. I owe a debt of gratitude to the individuals who have been named earlier in this Preface. In addition, as I have attended advanced EMG workshops, I have benefited from exposure to my peers in this specialty area. Many ideas and peer suggestions have been incorporated into this beginners' text. My years of work at the US Public Health Services, Division of Hospitals and Clinics, provided an excellent opportunity for developing the materials in this book and practicing in this clinical specialty area. I hope that users and readers of this book will find it helpful in developing beginning skills in this important area of clinical practice.

—John L. Echternach, EdD, PT, ECS, FAPTA

chapter 1

Instrumentation

OBJECTIVES

At the end of this unit of study the reader will be able to:

✦ Define and describe the basic principles of clinical electromyography.

✦ Describe the basic instrumentation required for EMG and NCV studies.

✦ Operate the equipment to demonstrate surface EMG potentials.

✦ Demonstrate a motor action potential by stimulation of a motor nerve.

✦ Explain the various operations the equipment performs and describe the functions of the controls on the front panel of the EMG machine.

✦ Define several reasons why artifacts may appear on the oscilloscope.

✦ Carry out a very basic troubleshooting approach to equipment failure.

Introduction

Clinical electromyography can only be performed by using needle electrodes so that the recording of electrical activity is from within the muscle being examined. Spontaneous activity cannot be recorded with surface electrodes. The unit of activity in clinical electromyography is based primarily on the study of individual motor units. This emphasis on motor unit activity that is individual in nature can be only studied by the use of needle electrodes. The reason for emphasizing this method of studying muscle activity is so that readers will not be confused when comparing clinical electromyographic studies with other uses of electromyography.

Studies of muscle activity using surface, as well as indwelling electrodes, have been done by those interested in kinesiologic analysis of muscle. As motor analysis becomes of greater importance in the clinical environment, increased use of electromyographic techniques for this clinical purpose has occurred.

Electromyography has also been used in a variety of biofeedback applications that have used surface electrodes. These applications have been used as adjuncts to treatment programs aimed at increasing or decreasing muscle activity, permitting patients to gain greater control over their muscle activity.

Electromyography may be defined as the study of the intrinsic electrical activity of muscle. It is based primarily on lower motor neuron phenomena. Electromyography, as used clinically, is most useful in studying anterior horn cell, nerve root, plexus, peripheral nerve, and primary muscle disorders. There are some interesting relationships relating electromyography to upper motor neuron problems, but, for the beginning electromyographer, this is theoretical and does not have a direct relationship to the clinical problems most often seen. In electromyography we speak of studying the characteristics of the different observable potentials. There are five characteristics that can be described for any electromyographic potential (Figures 1-1 and 1-2):

1. *Voltage* or amplitude of the response. This is a way of measuring the size of the potential from peak to peak. This measurement is in microvolts (μV) or millivolts (mV).

2. *Duration* is a measurement of how long it takes for the individual potential to complete itself; from the beginning of the first of its deviations (phases) from the baseline to the last deviation and back to the base line. This measurement is expressed in milliseconds (ms).

3. *Waveforms* are electromyographic potentials that may be monophasic, biphasic, etc. This describes the number of deviations (phases) from the baseline that the potential makes. Waveforms are described as one less than the number of crossings (eg, biphasic potential has three contacts/crossings of base line).

4. *Frequency* is a description of how often the potential occurs within a certain time frame, and is usually expressed as some number per second.

5. *Sound* is important because EMG potentials are displayed not only visually but can also be heard on a loud speaker, and their individual sound characteristics can be used in determining what type of electromyographic potential is being displayed.

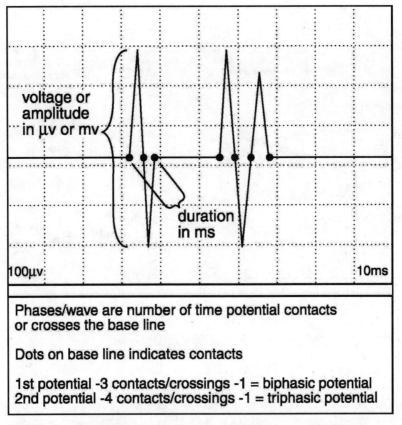

Figure 1-1. Illustration of EMG waveform characteristics of voltage (amplitude), duration, and phases.

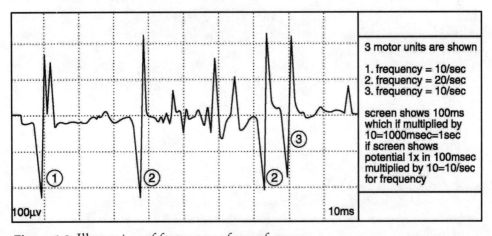

Figure 1-2. Illustration of frequency of waveforms.

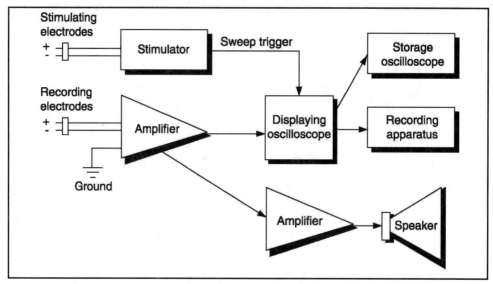

Figure 1-3. Basic components of an electromyograph.

Instrumentation

The basic features of the typical EMG are shown in Figure 1-3. Electrodes pick up the action potential that is conditioned by a preamplifier before being "magnified" by an amplifier. From the amplifier the signal is led to the monitoring and display portions of the instrument: (a) an oscilloscope (screen) to permit immediate display and visual monitoring of the potentials, (b) an audio amplifier and speaker to allow acoustic monitoring of the potentials, and (c) a recorder for permanent recording of the potentials. A stimulator (d) is necessary for performance of conduction velocities . The stimulator is electronically isolated and synchronized with the trace of the oscilloscope.

Three electrode components are necessary for EMG and NCV testing:

1. A *ground electrode* for reducing extraneous noise and interference

2. A *pick-up* or *recording electrode* (the negative electrode)

3. A *reference electrode* (the positive electrode)

The assignment of the designation of negative and positive to recording and reference electrodes is a convention used in practice and does not imply the possession of a charge by the electrode. There are a number of different types of electrode systems in which the three above components may be found (Figure 1-4).

Surface electrodes are composed of two metal discs with attached lead off wires. One disc is the recording electrode, the other the reference electrode. These discs may be embedded in a plastic block or be attached to separate wires to allow for flexible placement. Surface electrodes permit recording of the electrical activity of muscle but are not capable of recording a single motor unit or the short duration potentials caused by spontaneous activity in muscle. Surface electrodes are routinely used

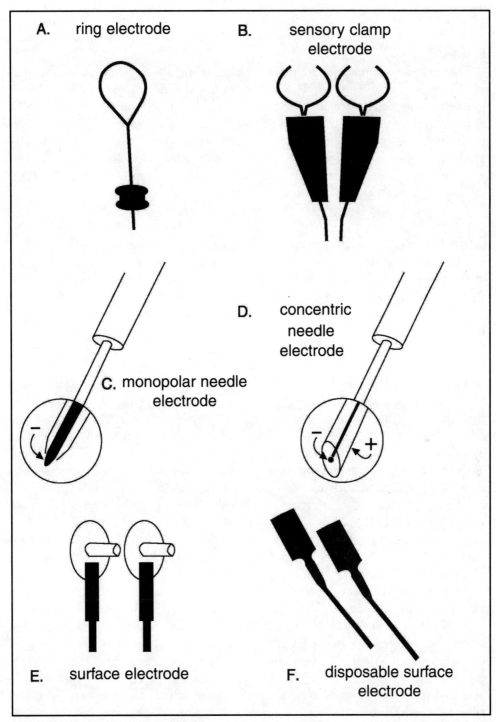

Figure 1-4. Examples of typical electrodes used in electromyography and nerve conduction studies.

for motor nerve conduction studies because they record the summated compound potential of many motor units instead of individual ones and compound sensory potentials.

Coaxial (concentric) needle electrodes allow recording directly from within the muscle. They consist of a platinum wire that is located centrally inside a hypodermic needle but completely insulated from it. The bare tip of the internal component acts as the recording electrode while the outside of the needle acts as the reference electrode. Both the internal wire and outside cannula are connected to the preamplifier input terminals. This type of electrode is used routinely for EMG studies because it is able to adequately record individual motor units as well as low-amplitude, short-duration potentials arising within muscle tissue.

A separate *ground electrode* usually consists of a large disc electrode affixed to the skin.

Triaxial (bipolar) needle electrodes are similar to concentric electrodes except that two platinum wires are embedded in the hypodermic needle, necessitating a larger diameter needle, and are therefore more painful upon insertion through the skin than other electrodes. Each wire inside is connected to the preamplifier input and the cannula becomes the ground; therefore, no separate surface ground electrode is necessary.

Monopolar needle electrodes are usually constructed from a stainless steel wire or needle sharpened to a pointed tip and then insulated with Teflon (Dupont, Wilmington, Del) except for the very tip. Monopolar electrodes are thinner than other needle electrodes and the Teflon coating reduces resistance to movement through tissues, making it less painful during insertion through the skin than the other types of needle electrodes. It is necessary to use another needle or a surface electrode as a reference electrode.

Recording electrodes pick up bioelectric potentials as well as interference signals. A preamplifier placed fairly close to the recording electrodes serves the purpose of reducing the amount of interference signal and enhancing the bioelectric potential. This amplifier is called a *differential amplifier*.

Earlier I alluded to the fact that the input signal is recorded from both a recording and a reference electrode, which means the differential amplifier has two sources of input. The differential amplifier amplifies differences that exist in the signals from the two inputs; however, it rejects signals that are common to both inputs. The signals that are common to both inputs are generally the unwanted signals from interference. The ability of an amplifier to reject these unwanted signals is called *common mode rejection*. The ability of an amplifier to reject these common mode signals is usually indicated by a term called the *common mode rejection ratio*. The higher this ratio, the greater the ability of the amplifier to reject the common mode potentials (see Appendix A for a definition of differential amplifiers and common mode rejection).

Once the signal has been processed, the signal from the preamplifier must be amplified further before it can be satisfactorily displayed and recorded. A related concept to the amplification of the bioelectric potentials of interest is the concept of gain. *Gain* may be defined as the ratio of the amplifier's output to its input signal. The concept of gain by an amplifier is related to a specific function of the EMG apparatus, which is termed sensitivity. *Sensitivity* is the ratio of the input voltage to the size of the deflection that is seen on the visual display of the oscilloscope. This deflection occurs vertically and can be expressed in mV or µV per division. *Amplitude of potentials* is measured by the use of the concept of sensitivity; however, the three terms are often used interchangeably in the description of a potential. That is, gain, sensitivity, and amplitude are all related.

Another related concept is that of *filter settings*. Differential amplifiers have both low- and high-frequency cutoff points. Basically, a high-frequency filter limits the higher frequencies from being recorded but allows lower frequencies to pass through and be recorded. A low-frequency filter, then, does the opposite; it keeps low frequencies from being observed but permits the higher frequencies to pass through, to be recorded. Commercially available instruments consist of variable high- and low-frequency filter systems that can be adjusted by the examiner to optimize the frequency content of the bioelectric potentials that are of interest. The use of the proper high- and low- frequency filter combinations improves the frequency content of the signal and limits undesired noise. Many times on modern equipment, the high and low frequency settings are chosen by the manufacturer and entered into the machine. These frequency settings can be altered by the clinician if the clinician desires. An example of frequency settings for filtration of the signal would be for needle EMG; these settings would be from 20 MHz to 10 kHz. Compare this to a typical setting for motor nerve conduction studies, which would be from 2 Hz to 10 kHz. As noted previously, commercial apparatus will allow the examiner to either choose the frequency settings or they will be preset, and the clinician needs to confirm what the settings are and change them for special applications when necessary.

Sometimes the biological potential being recorded is extremely small compared to the surrounding noise from other sources of electrical activity. In the course of performing conduction studies, sensory potentials are among the smallest potentials that are recorded. The use of *averaging* greatly enhances the possibility of capturing these very small potentials. When one uses an averager, the purpose is to improve the signal amplitude compared to all the surrounding noise that is being generated. In other words, one wishes to improve the signal-to-noise ratio. Generally speaking, the averager permits the examiner to pick a preselected number of traces that will be averaged. The examiner can then stimulate the nerve being studied the preselected number of times and display a summated trace on the oscilloscope. This process has excluded much of the unwanted noise and enhanced the signal to be examined as much as possible (see Appendix A for the definition of this process, see Appendix B for technical terms related to apparatus for EMG and evoked potential [EP] measurements).

Bibliography

Aminoff MJ. Electrodiagnostic apparatus. In: Aminoff MJ, ed. *Electromyography in Clinical Practice*. 3rd ed. NY: Churchill-Livingstone; 1998:45-62.

Dimitru D. Instrumentation. In: Dimitru D, ed. *Electrodiagnostic Medicine*. Philadelphia, Pa: Hanley & Belfus, Inc; 1995: 65-92.

King JC. Basic electricity primer. In: Dimitru D. ed. *Electrodiagnostic Medicine*. Philadelphia, Pa: Hanley and Belfus; 1995:93-107.

Oh S. Basic components of electromyography instruments. In: Oh S, ed. *Clinical Electromyography: Nerve Conduction Studies*. Baltimore, Md: University Park Press; 1984:47-64.

LABORATORY EXERCISE #1
Clinical EMG Techniques

Operation of EMG

1. Plug in the unit and turn it on.

2. Set up the unit according to the directions for EMG recording.

   (Sweep speed = 10 ms/div, sensitivity/gain: 200 (μV/div)

3. Locate and become familiar with the following controls (if available):
   A. On-off switch—Power control
   B. Oscilloscope/screen controls
   C. Intensity control or brightness*
   D. Focus*
   E. Vertical position adjustment*
   F. Horizontal position adjustment*
   G. Filters
   H. Timing signal
   I. Audio-speaker control
   J. Storage mode and/or recording method
   K. Conduction time marker (cursors)
   These functions are usually automatic

   There is a logical grouping of controls on the front panel or keyboard. Generally, if knobs are used, clockwise rotation of controls increases the intensity (sensitivity) of the event being monitored, and counter-clockwise rotation decreases it. Many models have buttons or microprocessor keys instead of knobs.

4. Two characteristics of the visual display (trace) must be adjusted frequently for effective testing. These are the horizontal control (sweep speed/time base) and the vertical control (sensitivity/amplitude/gain). Starting with the sweep speed at its longest setting (eg, the lowest number), adjust it through its complete range. Observe the base line. Return to the usual EMG setting. Put a calibration signal on the screen/oscilloscope if your machine permits this. Starting with the sensitivity selector on the lowest setting, switch through its complete range. Note the change in the calibration signal (the calibration of an EMG unit should be checked regularly and adjusted when necessary).

Surface Recording of Muscle Potentials (Biofeedback)

1. Set up the EMG unit in EMG mode (use 200 µV sensitivity and 10 ms/div). After cleansing the skin, apply a pair of surface electrodes to the abductor pollicis brevis muscle. Keep the electrodes at least 2 cm apart. Put a ground electrode on a nearby proximal bony prominence (eg, dorsum of hand or radial styloid).

   A. Switch the preamplifier to the patient position. Observe the oscilloscope when the muscle is relaxed, contracting slightly and contracting maximally.

   B. Vary the sweep speed (time/division). How does this change the displayed activity?

   C. Vary the vertical sensitivity (volt/division). How does this change the action potentials?

   D. Find a position where your subject can relax completely. Use a time base setting that permits you to roughly estimate the amplitude of the interference pattern.

2. To demonstrate the consequences of poor technique, perform the following in sequence:

   A. Remove the ground electrode.

   B. Lift one electrode from the muscle while it is contracting.

   C. Shake the lead wires vigorously.

   D. Place a line of electrode gel between both electrodes, then contract the muscle.

   E. Place the electrodes on the opposite thumb. Do not wash the skin or use electrode paste.

Nerve Conduction Velocity Determination

1. Set up the unit in the motor NCV mode (2 mV/div, 2 or 5 ms/div). Place two surface electrodes on the abductor digiti minimi. Switch the preamplifier to the patient position. Place the ground electrode on the dorsum of the hand. Set up the stimulator unit with a repetition rate of 1 pulse/second rate of stimulation with a pulse duration of 0.1 ms and the intensity at 0.

   Always return intensity to 0 before placing stimulator on skin.

   A. Place stimulator over the ulnar nerve at the wrist (next to the tendon of the flexor carpi ulnaris muscle).

   B. Gradually increase the stimulus until an evoked response is observed (compound muscle action potential [CMAP]). Increase the intensity of the stimulus until the response is maximal and further increases in stimulus intensity. Do not increase the amplitude of the waveform. This is a supramaximal stimulus. Note the characteristics of the evoked potential (see Figure 2-1).

C. Within the limits of tolerance of your subject, observe changes in the evoked waveform when you:

   a. Vary the voltage from minimal to supramaximal.

   b. Vary the vertical sensitivity (volts/div).

   c. Vary the sweep speed (time/div).

   d. Vary the duration of the stimulus from 0.1 to 0.5 ms.

   e. Vary the rate of stimulation from 0.5 to 5 pps.

Additional Equipment

1. Explore additional features of the instrumentation with which you are working:

   A. Storage methods

   B. Recording system, paper printout

   C. Foot controls

   D. Averager

Clean and return all equipment to the place where you found it. Leave the laboratory neat and ready for the next group.

SOURCES OF ELECTRICAL INTERFERENCE OR ARTIFACT

✧ Dirty electrodes

✧ Broken electrode lead wires (plus ground wire)

✧ Electrode wire movement

✧ Poor ground electrode location

✧ Incorrect connection of electrodes at input box

✧ Electrode paste bridging between ground and stimulating electrode

✧ Power cords in wall receptacles nearby

✧ Poor apparatus grounding

✧ Fluorescent lights

✧ Electronic dimmers

✧ Intermittent power line load

✧ Diathermy, radio or TV nearby

✧ Ungrounded power tools (drills, etc) operating nearby

General Troubleshooting Checklist

1. Check if AC power is applied: Is the unit plugged in? Are the On and Off switches on? Is the preamplifier switched to the on or patient position?

2. Inspect for blown fuse, loose wires, burned-out components (use your sense of smell).

3. Trace the major circuit components to identify the potential area of trouble:

   A. Erratic signals are usually loose connections of leads or interference from another electronic source.

   B. Noisy signal results at high gain from radiated noise (fluorescent lights) or internal noise from the instrument.

   C. If you don't know what you're doing, don't do it!

Review Questions

1. What are the basic instrumentation requirements for performing EMG and NCV studies?

2. What are the typical electrodes needed to perform a motor NCV?

3. What does the action potential recorded by the surface electrode represent when it is the result of muscle contraction? When is it the result of nerve stimulation?

4. What are the functions of the following controls of an EMG?
    a. time/div
    b. volts/div
    c. repetition rate
    d. stimulus duration
    e. averager
    f. cursor
    g. audio control

5. Briefly describe four causes of electrical artifact. Explain the source of each.

6. In what situations would a high and low setting be used for the "filters?"

Nerve Conduction Studies

OBJECTIVES

At the end of this unit of study the reader will be able to:

✧ Describe the basic characteristics and principles of nerve conduction velocity testing.

✧ Demonstrate the general procedures for performing motor and sensory conduction studies.

✧ Perform motor conduction studies of the peroneal and tibial nerves of the lower extremities.

✧ Perform motor conduction studies of the ulnar and median nerves of the upper extremities.

✧ Perform, with assistance, motor conduction studies of the radial, musculocutaneous, facial, and femoral nerves.

✧ Perform sensory conduction studies of the ulnar, median, sural, and superficial peroneal nerves.

✧ Describe the normal values for each of the above-described nerves.

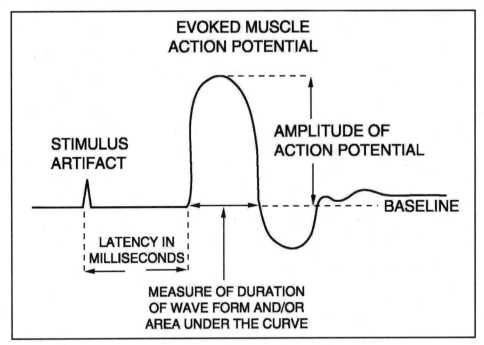

Figure 2-1. Elements of the evoked muscle action potential.

Nerve Conduction Study Characteristics

The characteristics, which may be measured by means of nerve conduction studies (NCS), are as follows (Figure 2-1):

1. *Latency* is the time lapse delay, in milliseconds (ms) from the introduction of the stimulus (stimulus artifact) to its evoked response recorded by the paired recording and reference electrodes.

2. *Conduction velocity* is the rate in meters per second (m/sec) at which an impulse (action potential) travels along a nerve segment.

3. *Amplitude* is the magnitude in microvolts (µV) or millivolts (mV) recorded by the active and reference electrodes and displayed on the oscilloscope as a vertical displacement of the baseline. Measured from baseline to peak of the negative waveform of motor nerve potentials and peak to peak for sensory nerve potentials.

4. *Waveform* is the shape and number of phases of the response recorded by the recording electrodes and displayed on the oscilloscope.

5. *Duration* is the time in milliseconds it takes for the negative phase of the evoked potential to return to the baseline.

Basic Principles in
Nerve Conduction Velocity Testing

Motor conduction velocity is not constant along the entire length of the nerve. As an impulse approaches the distal portion of a nerve where terminal branching occurs, it is slowed. It is further delayed as it traverses the myoneural junction. In order to obtain an accurate evaluation of nerve impulse (action potential) velocity, it is necessary to eliminate the terminal slowing and myoneural junction transmission by providing electrical stimulation at two separate points along the nerve, proximal to the terminal branching. Two action potentials are obtained representing these two points of stimulation. The distance along the extremity between the two points of stimulation measured in millimeters is divided by the time required for the nerve impulse to traverse this distance. This time is obtained by subtracting the time (T1) of the more distal latency from the proximal (T2) latency. Calculation of nerve conduction velocity is described by the formula below.

CALCULATION OF NERVE CONDUCTION VELOCITY

$$\text{NCV (m/sec)} = \frac{D = (\text{millimeters})(\text{meters})}{T2\text{-}T1\ (\text{milliseconds})(\text{seconds})}$$

Key:

NCV = Nerve conduction velocity

D = Distance between proximal and more distal stimulation sites measured between negative poles (measured in millimeters)

T2 = Latency at proximal stimulation site

T1 = Latency at distal stimulation site

Using the median nerve as an example, we can compute the conduction velocity of the median nerve, where the latency obtained on stimulating the median nerve at the wrist and recording from the abductor pollicis brevis is 3 ms (T1) and the latency stimulating at the medial aspect of the elbow over the median nerve is 8 ms (T2). The measurement between these two sites of stimulation is 300 mm (D). Entering this information into the equation above would yield:

$$\text{NCV (m/sec)} = \frac{300\text{mm}}{8\ \text{ms} - 3\ \text{ms}} = 60\ \text{m/sec}$$

Because the units of measure are equivalent, we can directly use the answer as m/sec. If the distance (D) measurement is in centimeters, then the resulting answer must be multiplied by 10 to convert to m/sec.

This procedure can be used on any segment of nerve that is anatomically possible to stimulate. For example, NCV studies can be performed on the median nerve from the supraclavicular area to the wrist.

When it is necessary to test a segment of nerve in which it is not anatomically feasible to stimulate at two points, the latency is obtained. Despite the fact that this measurement includes the terminal branching and the myoneural junction, this can be a very useful measurement when comparing obtained results with established latency norms and normal nerves of the same subject. Examples of nerves where latency measurements are used are the facial nerve in Bell's palsy and the median nerve in carpal tunnel syndrome.

Impulses do not travel along individual nerve fibers at the same rate, nor do nerve fibers have the same threshold to electrical stimulation. When a nerve is stimulated and the impulse is propagated along the nerve to the muscle, the evoked action potential that is elicited is a summation of impulses of many nerve fibers that travel at different rates. The fastest fibers contribute to the first part of the evoked action potential where it first leaves the baseline. The latency is, therefore, a measurement of the fastest conducting fibers within the nerve. It is critical that the point of measurement (the first point of deflection of the action potential) is completely consistent each time the nerve is stimulated along its course, ensuring accuracy. In order to consistently ensure stimulation of all nerve fibers, a supramaximal stimulus is necessary when performing NCV studies. This eliminates the possibility of measuring the speed of different nerve fibers at different stimulation points along the nerve. To further verify that the same nerve fibers are being stimulated, the evoked action potential should be observed. It should have the same approximate parameters (ie, amplitude, shape, and duration) each time the nerve is stimulated.

Sensory Nerve Conduction Testing

When a nerve is stimulated, the impulse is propagated proximally as well as distally. Sensory conduction velocity may be measured by recording evoked sensory potentials along the course of the nerve. Two methods may be used. The *orthodromic method* refers to impulse propagation along axons in the normal or physiologic direction of sensory conduction (eg, distal to proximal). With this method, the nerve is stimulated at a distal point and the potentials are recorded at a proximal point along the course of the nerve. The *antidromic method* is opposite of the orthodromic (ie, opposite the normal or physiologic sensory nerve direction of propagation). The nerve trunk is stimulated at proximal points and the potential recorded at a distal point in the sensory area.

Sensory nerve potentials are much smaller than motor potential; some may be as low as 5 µV or smaller. When recording sensory NCV, precision in technique and careful attention to grounding is essential.

Sensory conduction testing may be a more sensitive measure in determination of early abnormalities of peripheral neuropathy than motor NCVs.

The nerves most easily tested for sensory NCV are the median and ulnar nerves, although many other nerves such as the radial, sural, and superficial peroneal nerves can be tested.

GENERAL PROCEDURE

The first step for performing motor and sensory nerve conduction velocities is to review all charts and records available for the patient, especially sensory and motor function examinations. Then, introduce yourself to the patient and perform any further examination procedures deemed necessary to obtain the information firsthand. There is no substitute for a thorough examination of the patient prior to testing.

Turn on the electromyograph and check to be certain that the recording method available is functioning properly. Explain the nature of the study to the patient, position the patient comfortably, expose the part(s) to be tested, and drape the patient appropriately.

Check that the stimulator and preamplifier electrode input box are both properly plugged into the machine.

Cleanse the skin area with an alcohol swab and wipe dry with gauze where recording, ground, and stimulating electrodes are to be placed. To further reduce skin resistance, if necessary, rub the skin gently with very fine sandpaper and then cleanse the skin with alcohol and dry with gauze to remove surface oils and dry skin.

After putting a small amount of electrode gel on the recording electrode and ground, position:

1. Motor recording electrodes:
    A. Place the recording (negative) disc electrode over the belly of the muscle. Secure tightly—nonallergic, "elastic" tape works well for securing surface electrodes.
    B. Place the reference disc electrode over the muscle tendon, distal to the position of the recording electrode. Secure tightly.

2. Sensory recording electrodes:
    A. Place the recording (negative) flexible ring electrode around the mid-proximal phalanx of a digit.
    B. Place the reference (positive) flexible ring electrode around the distal phalanx distal to the recording electrode by 2 cm or more.

3. Ground:
    A. For sensory and motor NCVs place the ground electrode over a bony area (eg, dorsum of hand) as close to the recording electrodes as possible.

Plug the recording, reference, and ground electrodes into the jacks of the preamplifier.

Check to be certain that the recording electrodes are positioned and functioning properly. One way this may be accomplished for motor studies is to set the function to EMG and ask the patient to contract the muscle if possible. EMG potentials should be displayed if the patient can contract the muscle.

Adjust the machine setting:

1. For motor nerves 2 (or 5) ms/div, 2 (or 5) mV/div; sensory nerves 2 ms/div, 10 or 20 µV/div. Set stimulator at 0.1/ms duration and at a rate of 1 pps. A 0.05 setting may be used for sensory testing.

2. Set audio volume at appropriate level.

A suggested procedure for doing a motor NCV is, with the intensity set at zero, put a small amount of electrode gel on the tips of the stimulating electrodes and proceed as follows:

1. Motor procedure:

   A. Palpate the nerve at the point chosen as the most distal of the series of nerve stimulation sites.

   B. At the chosen sites, place the negative (black) electrode distally, and the positive (red) electrode proximally over the nerve.

   C. Gradually begin to increase the intensity of stimulus until the patient becomes accustomed to the current, then increase the current gradually to a supramaximal level. Always use a supramaximal stimulus for stimulation at all additional sites. To make the patient comfortable, repeat the above procedure at each site.

   D. Listen for the characteristic "thudding sound" on the audio speaker, indicating that you are "solidly" over the nerve and observe the muscle movement produced.

   E. Store the response and use the latency indicator (cursor) to mark the initial point of take-off of the muscle action potential (CMAP) or M-response from the baseline and concurrently determine the amplitude of the negative waveform from baseline to peak.

   F. Record the amplitude, latency, and stored response. Wipe the electrode gel from patient and mark the site where the cathode of the stimulator was placed. A felt-tip pen works well for marking stimulation sites.

   G. Stimulate the nerve again, this time at a more proximal stimulation site. Follow the procedure outlined above.

   H. If you wish to stimulate the same nerve at other sites, follow the procedure presented above.

   I. Record the patient's name, date of test, nerve tested, sites of stimulation, stimulus duration and sensitivity (amplitude), and time base setting per tracing (most equipment will do this automatically).

   J. Measure the distance in centimeters or millimeters (1 cm = 10 mm) between each stimulation site as marked on the patient using a good quality steel metric tape measure. If uneven surface contours are a concern, a caliper can be used to measure between stimulation sites.

2. Sensory procedure:

   A. Use the same basic procedure as outlined for the motor procedure.

   B. Usually the motor NCV is performed before the sensory study and, if so, you may use the same stimulation site(s) as used for the motor nerve conduction if you are using the antidromic method.

   C. Often, only a distal sensory latency is performed on sensory nerves, but as with the motor nerve, a series of stimulation sites in a distal-proximal direction may be used for antidromic studies. As you move the stimulation site proximally, the amplitude of the sensory potential may drop.

Calculate the NCV using the formula described previously. Sensory NCVs can be calculated directly by measuring the distance from the site of simulation to the recording electrode, since there is no motor end-plate or other intervening structure.

Bibliography

Aminoff MJ. Electromyography in clinical practice. In: Aminoff MJ, ed. *Nerve Conduction Studies: Basic Principles and Pathologic Correlations.* 3rd ed. New York: Churchill Livingstone; 1998: 113-145.

Dimitru D. Nerve conduction studies. In: Dimitru D, ed. *Electrodiagnostic Medicine.* Philadelphia, Pa: Hanley and Belfus; 1995: 111-175.

Echternach JL. The use of conduction velocity measurements as an evaluation tool. In: Wolf SL, ed. *Electrotherapy.* New York: Churchill Livingstone; 1981.

Echternach JL. Measurement issues in nerve conduction velocity and electromyographic testing. In: Rothstein JM, ed. *Measurement in Physical Therapy.* New York: Churchill Livingstone; 1985.

Eddy JG, Snyder-Mackler L. Clinical electrophysiologic testing. In: Robinson A, Snyder-Mackler L, eds. *Clinical Electrophysiology.* 2nd ed. Baltimore, Md: Williams and Wilkins; 1998.

Kimura J. *Electrodiagnosis in Diseases of Nerve and Muscle.* 2nd ed. Philadelphia, Pa: FA Davis; 1989.

Liveson JA. Localized processes. In: Liveson JA, ed. *Peripheral Neurology: Case Studies in Electrodiagnosis.* 2nd ed. Philadelphia, Pa: FA Davis; 1991.

Nelson C. Electrical evaluation of nerve and muscle excitability. In: Gersh MR, ed. *Electrotherapy in Rehabilitation.* Philadelphia, Pa: FA Davis; 1992.

Nestor D, Nelson RM. Electrophysiologic evaluation: an overview. In: Nelson RM, Hayes KW, Currier DP, eds. *Clinical Electrotherapy.* 2nd ed. Baltimore, Md: Williams and Wilkins; 1999.

Oh S. Nerve conduction techniques. In: Oh S, ed. *Clinical Electromyography: Nerve Conduction Studies.* Baltimore, Md: University Park Press; 1984:47-64.

Weber R. Nerve conduction studies. In: Johnson EW, Pease WS, eds. *Practical Electromyography.* 3rd ed. Baltimore, Md: Williams and Wilkins; 1997.

LABORATORY EXERCISE 2
Nerve Conduction

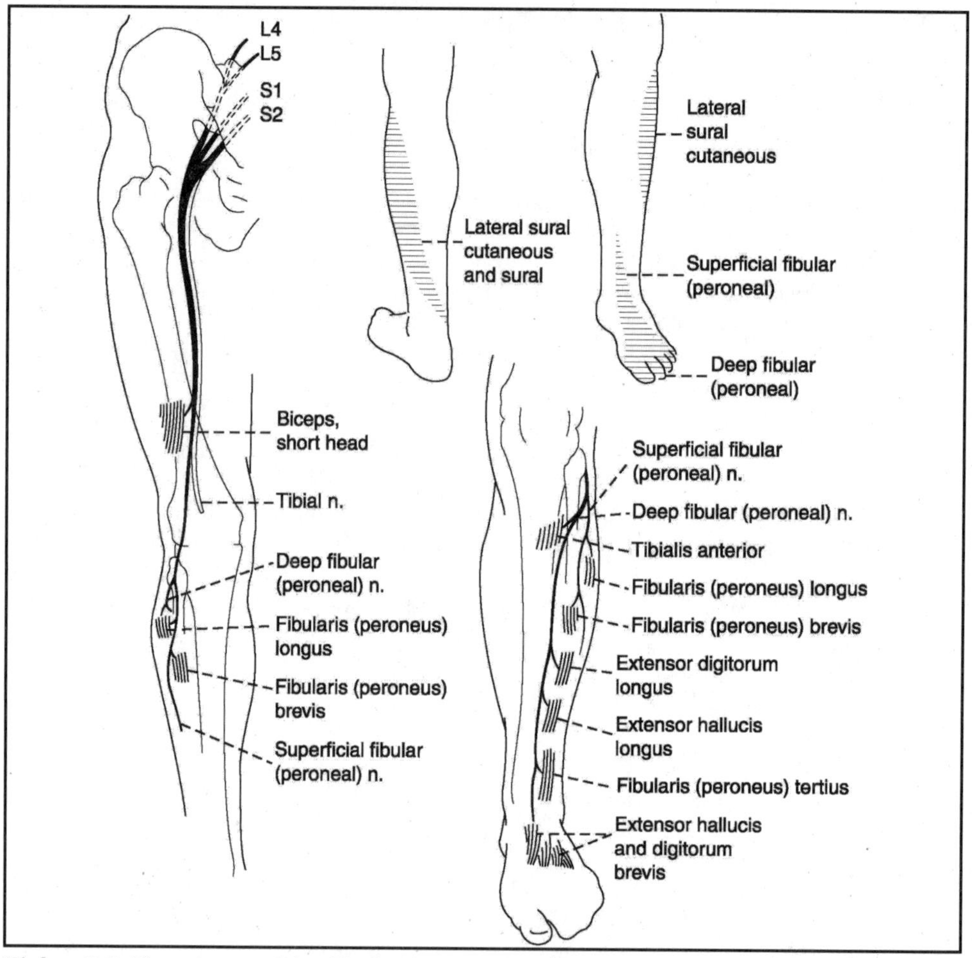

Figure 2-2. The course of the fibular (peroneal) nerve is shown, illustrating the motor and sensory distribution of the nerve.

OBJECTIVE

At the conclusion of this laboratory session the reader will be able to perform motor nerve conduction studies of the fibular (peroneal) and tibial nerves (Figure 2-2).

1. Set up EMG machine for motor nerve conduction velocity testing.

   A.   Sensitivity—2 mV/div (somewhere between 1 and 5 mV/div)

   B.   Sweep—2 (or 5) ms/div

   C.   Stimulus

      a.   Rate—1 pps (try other rates such as 2 pps,—see which you find most convenient)

      b.   Duration—0.1 ms

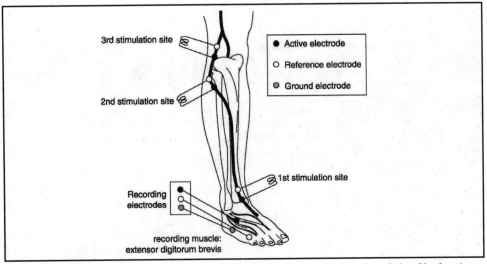

Figure 2-3. Sites of stimulation for motor nerve conduction study of the fibular (peroneal) nerve.

2. Subject positioning
    A. Fibular (peroneal)—supine (preferred) or sidelying
    B. Tibial—prone (preferred) or sidelying

3. Fibular (peroneal) nerve—electrode placement sites are shown in Figure 2-3, which also shows the sites of stimulation for a MNCV. Table 2-1 can be used for recording results.
    A. Recording electrode (negative)
        a. Muscle belly of extensor digitorum brevis (try stimulating with stimulating electrode to find the muscle)
    B. Reference (positive)
        a. Fifth toe extensor tendon or fifth metatarsal head
    C. Ground—lateral dorsum of foot, alternate sites: lower tibial shaft, calcaneus, or lateral malleolus
    D. Stimulating electrode placement sites: distal to proximal
        a. Anterior portion of ankle—between anterior tibialis and extension hallucis longus tendons, keep this segment at least 8 to10 cm from recording electrode
        b. Immediately inferior to head of fibula
        c. Posterolateral portion of popliteal fossa of posterior knee at least 10 cm above previous site

4. Tibial nerve—Figure 2-4 shows the motor and sensory distribution of the tibial nerve.

Table 2-1	FIBULAR (PERONEAL) NERVE							
		Latency (ms)		Distance (cm)		Amplitude (mV)		NCV (m/sec)
Anatomic Site	L	R	L	R	L	R	L	R
Anterior Ankle								
Fibular Head								
Posterior Knee								

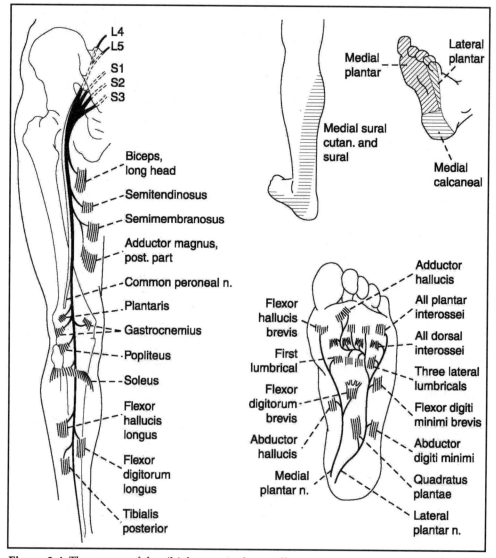

Figure 2-4. The course of the tibial nerve is shown illustrating the motor and sensory distribution of the nerve.

A. Recording electrodes (Figure 2-5 shows the sites of electrode placement and sites of simulation for MNCV of the tibial nerve)

    a. Medial plantar nerve—active electrode, use muscle belly of abductor hallucis (most commonly used for routine exam)

    b. Lateral plantar nerve—active electrode, use muscle belly of abductor digiti minimi

B. Reference

    a. Electrode at first metatarsal head (abductor hallucis)

    b. Electrode at fifth metatarsal head (abductor digiti minimi)

C. Ground—lateral malleolus, alternatives are lower tibial shaft or lateral dorsum of foot

D. Stimulating electrode placement sites

    a. Just proximal and posterior to medial malleolus (10 to 12 cm distance to recording electrode)

    b. Midpopliteal fossa of posterior knee

E. Record results—Table 2-2 can be used to record results.

5. Normal values

  A. Fibular (peroneal)—conduction velocity: 40 to 59 m/sec

  B. Distal latency: 2.4 to 6.0 ms

  C. Amplitude: 3 to 14 mV

  D. Tibial—conduction velocity: 40 to 59 m/sec

6. Distal latency to:

  A. Abductor hallucis brevis: 3.5 to 6.0 ms

  B. Abductor digiti minimi: 4.0 to 6.8 ms

  C. Amplitude: 3 to 15 mV

Distal latency values are meaningful for comparisons within the same extremity only when distances are equal.

Normal values are guidelines only. In each clinic this will vary somewhat depending on equipment and technique used. Normal values should be established from each clinic's experiences.

Additional normal values from *Clinical Electromyographies* by Shin and Oh are found in Tables 2-3 and 2-4.

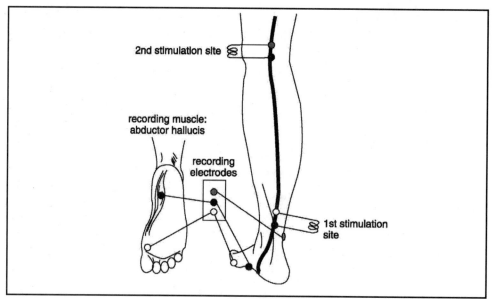

Figure 2-5. Sites of stimulation for motor nerve conduction study of the tibial nerve.

TIBIAL NERVE								
	Latency (ms)		Distance (cm)		Amplitude (mV)		NCV (m/sec)	
Anatomic Site	L	R	L	R	L	R	L	R
Medial Malleolus of Ankle								
Politeal Space—Knee								

Table 2-2

Table 2-3

PERONEAL MOTOR NERVE CONDUCTION

Parameter	Terminal Latency (msec)	NCV (m/sec) FibH-Ank	NCV (m/sec) PopF-FibH	CMAP Duration (msec)	CMAP Amplitude (mV)
Mean + SD	3.72 + 0.53	49.51 + 3.93	53.93 + 3.93	11.84 + 2.22	10.09 + 4.81
Normal limit	4.78	41.65	39.11	16.28	4.00

FibH-Ank = fibular head—ankle
PopF-FibH = popliteal fossa—fibular head
SD = standard deviation

Table 2-4

POSTERIOR TIBIAL MOTOR NERVE CONDUCTION

Parameter	Terminal Latency (ms)	NCV (m/sec) Fossa-Ankle (m/sec)	CMAP Duration (ms)	CMAP Amplitude (mV)
Mean + SD	3.85 + 0.63	49.83 + 4.60	12.30 + 3.26	19.06 + 7.23
Normal limit	5.11	40.63	18.82	5.00

LABORATORY EXERCISE 3
Nerve Conduction

OBJECTIVE

At the conclusion of this lab the reader will be able to perform motor nerve conduction studies of the ulnar and median nerves.

The course of the ulnar nerve is illustrated in Figure 2-6. Figure 2-7 illustrates the course of the median nerve. Use Tables 2-5 and 2-6 to record the results of this lab exercise.

1. Set up the EMG machine for motor nerve conduction velocity testing.
   A. Sensitivity—5 mV/div (somewhere between 2 and 5 mV/div)
   B. Sweep—2 (or 5) ms/div
   C. Stimulus
      a. Rate—1/sec
      b. Duration—0.1 ms
   D. Filters—MNCV—frequency response 2 Hz to 10 kHz

2. Position subject
   A. Supine
      a. Elbow 90-degree flexed and shoulder abducted to 90 degrees and externally rotated for the ulnar nerve
      b. Arm abducted to approximately 45 degrees at the shoulder with the elbow straight for the median nerve

3. Ulnar nerve-electrode placement (Figure 2-8 shows sites of electrode placement and sites of stimulation of the ulnar nerve. Figure 2-9 shows the details of the ulnar and median nerves of the hand)
   A. Recording electrode (negative)
      a. Muscle belly of abductor digiti minimi (ADM)
      b. Muscle belly of first dorsal interosseous (First DI) to the test deep branch of the ulnar nerve in hand
   B. Reference electrode (positive)
      a. Proximal phalanx of fifth digit-volar surface
      b. Proximal phalanx of thumb-dorsal surface
   C. Ground
      a. Dorsum of hand
   D. Stimulating electrode placement sites

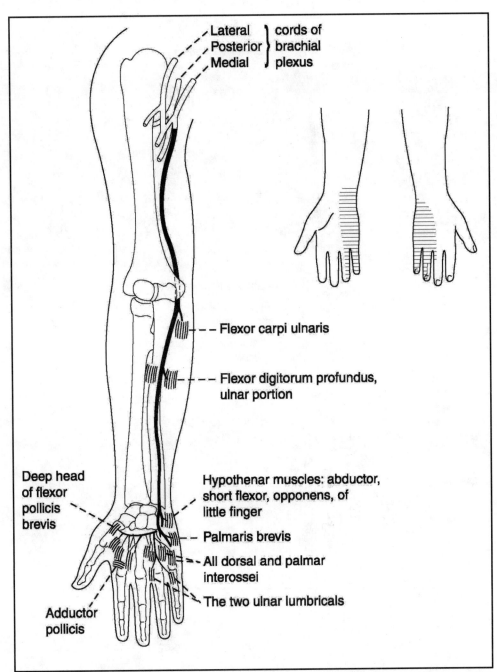

Figure 2-6. The course of the ulnar nerve is shown illustrating the motor and sensory distribution of the nerve.

a. Wrist, next to the tendon of the flexor carpi ulnaris—8 cm proximal measured from the recording electrode over the ADM

b. Approximately 2 cm below the medial epicondyle—over the dorsal surface of the forearm

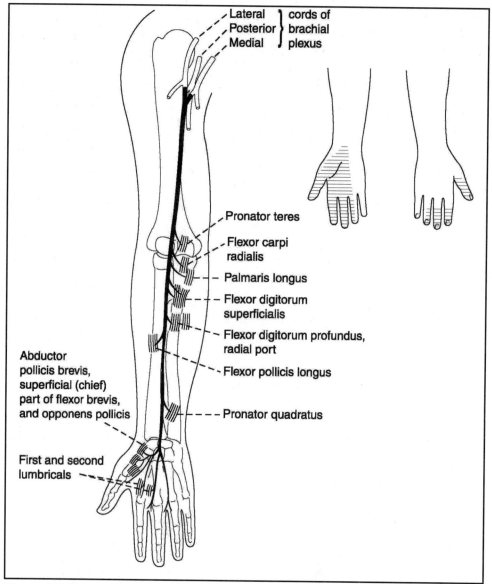

Figure 2-7. Illustration showing the course of the median nerve.

    c. 10 cm or more proximal to above site—over the medial aspect of the arm

    d. 10 cm or more proximal to above elbow site high on the medial aspect of the arm or axilla

4. Median nerve—electrode placement (Figure 2-10 shows the sites for electrode placement and sites of stimulation for the median nerve)

    A. Recording electrode (negative)

        a. Muscle belly of abductor pollicis brevis (APB)

Table 2-5

ULNAR NERVE

Anatomic Site	Latency (ms)		Distance (cm)		Amplitude (mV)		NCV (m/sec)	
	L	R	L	R	L	R	L	R
Wrist								
Below Elbow								
Above Elbow								
Upper Arm								

Table 2-6

MEDIAN NERVE

Anatomic Site	Latency (ms)		Distance (cm)		Amplitude (mV)		NCV (m/sec)	
	L	R	L	R	L	R	L	R
Wrist								
Elbow								
Upper Arm								

B. Reference electrode (positive)

    a. Proximal phalanx of thumb, volar surface

C. Ground

    a. Dorsum of hand

D. Stimulating electrode placement sites

    a. Wrist—between tendons of the flexor carpi radialis and palmaris tongue—8 cm proximal measured from the recording electrode

    b. Elbow—medial to the biceps tendon and just proximal to the volar surface of the medial epicondyle

    c. Proximal upper arm—medial aspect—or axilla

5. Normal values—conduction velocities and distal latencies (Tables 2-7 and 2-8)

    A. Ulnar nerve latency to ADM: 2.5 to 4.0 ms, latency to first DI (deep branch less than 1.5 ms greater than latency to ADM)

        a. Upper arm to above elbow: 55 to 65 m/sec

        b. Above elbow to below elbow: 50 to 60 m/sec

        c. Below elbow to wrist: 50 to 60 m/sec

        d. Amplitude: 4 to 14 mV

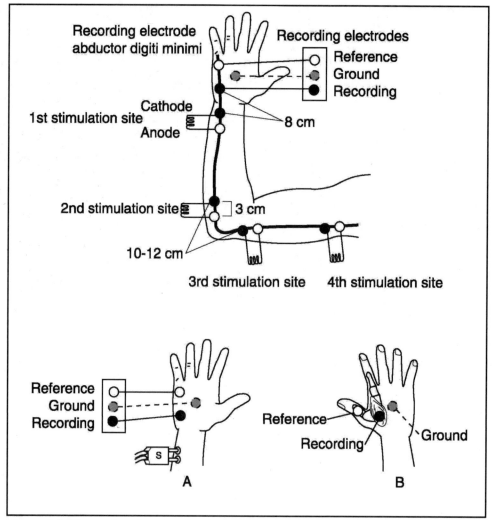

Figure 2-8. Illustration showing the sites of electrode placement and sites of stimulation of the ulnar nerve.

B. Median nerve

   a. Latency to APB: 2.7 to 4.0 ms

   b. Upper arm to elbow: 55 to 65 m/sec

   c. Elbow to wrist: 50 to 60 m/sec

   d. Amplitude: 4 to 14 mV

For both the ulnar and median nerves, the muscle action potential should be similar in waveform and amplitude at each stimulation site for each nerve. The waveforms for each nerve are distinctive. The ulnar waveform often has a mildly notched appearance as it rises to the peak amplitude.

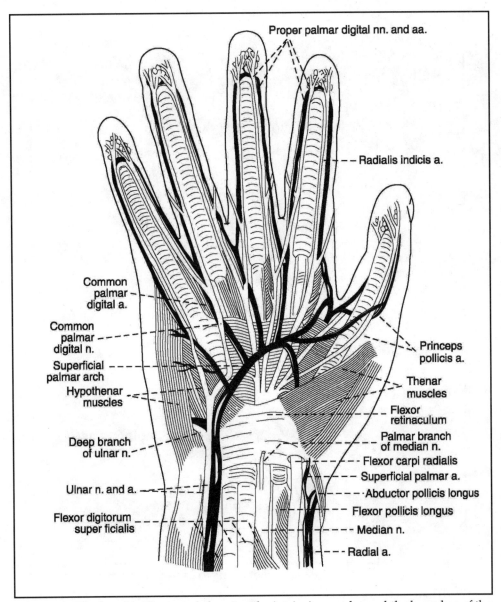

Figure 2-9. The hand is illustrated showing the intrinsic muscles and the branches of the ulnar and median nerves.

Care must be taken to guard against a volume conducted response to the nerve not being studied, especially in the upper arm sites. It is very easy to stimulate both nerves in this area, causing a change in waveform and amplitude that can be misleading. The same problem can occur when stimulating either nerve at the wrist.

When stimulating the ulnar nerve at the below elbow site, avoid stimulating too distally, because the ulnar nerve at this site enters the flexor carpi ulnaris muscle.

Care should be exercised in making measurements between points of stimulation of both nerves. Try to approximate the anatomic course of the nerve. This is especially important for both nerves at the wrist and the ulnar nerve across the elbow.

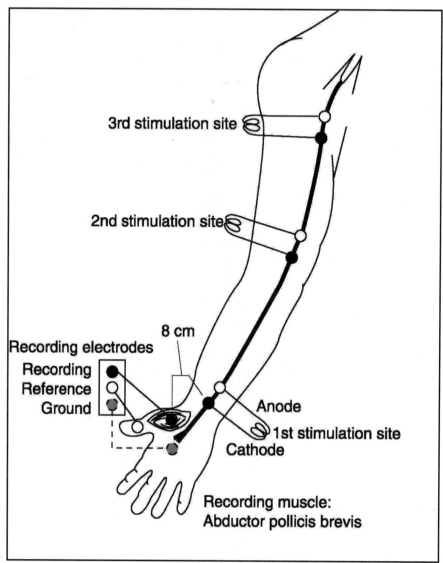

Figure 2-10. Sites of stimulation for motor nerve conduction study of the median nerve.

Case histories are presented at the end of this chapter that illustrate the usefulness of clinical electrophysiologic testing of these nerves. The electromyographic findings that accompany the nerve conduction information should be reviewed again after completing that part of the manual. Including the information here helps to demonstrate that by itself a nerve conduction study is unable to completely clarify a patient's condition. Both aspects of testing are needed for complete electrophysiologic understanding of a patient's condition.

Table 2-7

MEDIAN MOTOR NERVE CONDUCTION

Parameter	Terminal Latency (msec)	NCV (m/sec) Elbow Wrist	Axilla Elbow	CMAP Duration (msec)	Amplitude (mV)
Mean + SD	2.78 + 0.41	58.78 + 4.41	65.76 + 4.90	12.58 + 1.68	14.62 + 8.45
Normal Limit	3.60	49.96	55.96	15.94	5.00

Table 2-8

ULNAR MOTOR NERVE CONDUCTION

Parameter	Terminal Latency	NCV (m/sec) Elbow Wrist	Axilla Elbow	Erb's Point- Axilla	CMAP Duration (msec)	Amplitude (mV)
Mean + SD	2.03 + 0.24	61.16 + 5.27	63.33 + 5.47	68.36 + 5.07	13.43 + 1.61	11.49 + 2.51
Normal Limit	2.52	50.61	52.69	58.22	16.63	5.00

LABORATORY EXERCISE 4
Nerve Conduction Studies

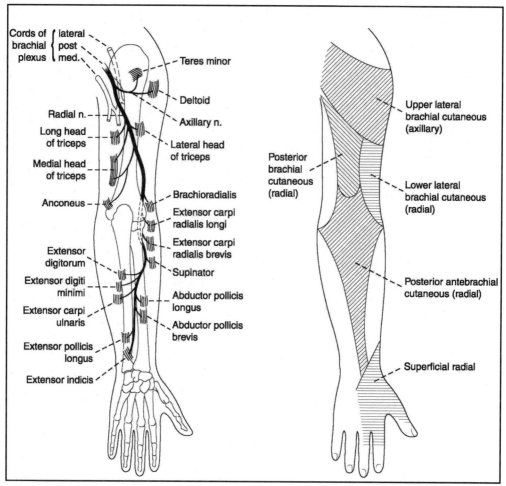

Figure 2-11. The course of the radial nerve is shown illustrating the motor and sensory distribution of the nerve.

OBJECTIVE

At the conclustion of this laboratory exercise, the reader will become familiar with the techniques for motor nerve conduction testing of less frequently tested nerves (radial, musculocutaneous, facial, and femoral nerves).

Figures 2-11 and 2-12 show the motor and sensory distribution of the radial and femoral nerves respectively. Record the results of this lab exercise using Tables 2-9, 2-10, and 2-11.

1. Set up equipment for a motor nerve conduction study as in Laboratory Exercises 2 and 3.

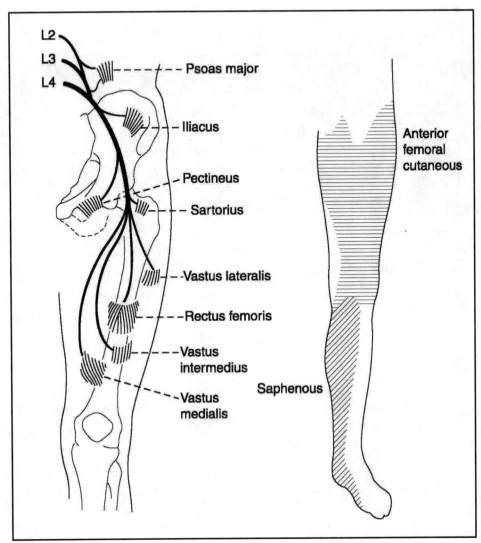

Figure 2-12. The course of the femoral nerve is shown illustrating the motor and sensory distribution.

Table 2-9

RADIAL NERVE

Anatomic Site	Latency (msec)		Distance (cm)		Amplitude (mV)		NCV (m/sec)	
	L	R	L	R	L	R	L	R
Forearm								
Elbow								
Lateral Arm								
Supraclavicular								

MUSCULOCUTANEOUS NERVE

Anatomic Site	Latency (ms)		Distance (cm)		Amplitude (mV)		NCV (m/sec)	
	L	R	L	R	L	R	L	R
Axilla								
Supraclavicular								
Facial Nerve								

Latency _____ ms to orbicularis oris (try latency to distance _____ ms ther sites such as frontalis muscle).

FEMORAL NERVE

Anatomic Site	Latency (msec)		Distance (cm)		Amplitude (mV)		NCV (m/sec)	
	L	R	L	R	L	R	L	R
Above Inguinal Lig								
Femoral Triangle								
Adductor Canal								

2. Position patient (supine)

3. Nerves to be examined:

A. Radial nerve (Figure 2-13 shows the electrode placement and sites of stimulation for the radial nerve)

a. Recording electrode (negative)

i. Extensor pollicis longus or brevis (surface electrode)

b. Reference electrode (positive)

i. Distal to the recording electrode over the tendon of the thumb extensors just above the radial styloid process

c. Ground electrode

i. Over the distal ulnar—between the recording and reference electrodes

d. Stimulation sites

i. Above the clavicle (Erb's point) (supraclavicular)

ii. Lateral aspect arm—10 cm or more above the lateral epicondyle (lateral arm)

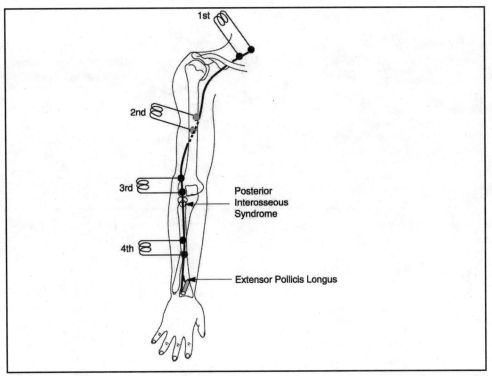

Figure 2-13. Illustration showing electrode placement and stimulation sites for the radial nerve.

    iii. Anticubital fossa, at the space between the border of the of brachioradialis muscle and the biceps tendon (elbow) (this site is used primarily when the patient has suspected compression of the posterior interosseus nerve in or near the radial tunnel)

    iv. Mid-dorsum of forearm, 8 cm above the recording electrode (forearm)

B. Musculocutaneous nerve

   a. Recording electrode

     i. Biceps—middle of the muscle belly area

   b. Reference electrode

     i. Distal portion of biceps—3 or 4 cm below the recording electrode

   c. Ground electrode

     i. Acromium process

   d. Stimulaton sites

     i. Above the clavicle (supraclavicular area)

     ii. Axilla—most proximal area of the anterior dome of the axilla

C. Facial nerve

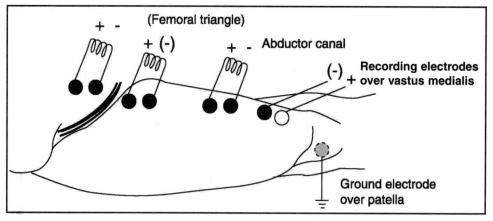

Figure 2-14. Sites of stimulation for motor nerve conduction study of the femoral nerve.

   a. Recording electrode

      i. Orbicularis oris (corner of the mouth) (can test different branches by placing electrodes over frontalis, orbicularis oculi, depressor anguli oris, etc)

   b. Reference electrode

      i. Two centimeters from recording electrode over the same muscle

   c. Stimulating electrodes

      i. Stylomastoid foramen (as facial nerve emerges at the lower edge of the ear)

   d. Ground

      i. Mandible at the angle of the mandible or forehead at hair line

  D. Femoral nerve (Figure 2-14 shows the sites for electrode placement and sites of stimulation for the femoral nerve)

   a. Recording electrode

      i. Vastus medialis at muscle belly

   b. Reference electrode

      i. Distal to the recording electrode by 3 cm (tendinous area)

   c. Ground

      i. Medial condyle of tibia or patella

   d. Stimulation sites

      i. Above the inguinal ligament—at least 6 cm above the femoral triangle, make distance as large as possible

      ii. Below inguinal ligament (femoral triangle)

      iii. Adductor canal (Hunter's canal)

4. Report results
5. Normal values
   A. Radial nerve
      a. Distal latency: 2.5 ms
      b. Amplitude: 3 to 9 mV
      c. Conduction velocity
         i. Elbow to forearm: 60 m/sec
         ii. Lateral arm to elbow: 65 m/sec
         iii. Supraclavicular to lateral arm: 70 m/sec
   B. Musculocutaneous nerve: 70 m/sec
      a. Distal latency: 2 to 4 ms
   C. Facial nerve
      a. Latency: 3.2 to 5.0 ms
   D. Femoral nerve
      a. Distal latency: 2 to 4 ms
      b. Latency difference above inguinal ligament to femoral triangle: less than 1.1 ms difference
      c. Conduction velocity
         i. Femoral triangle to adductor canal: 69 m/sec

LABORATORY EXERCISE 5
Sensory Nerve Conduction Velocity

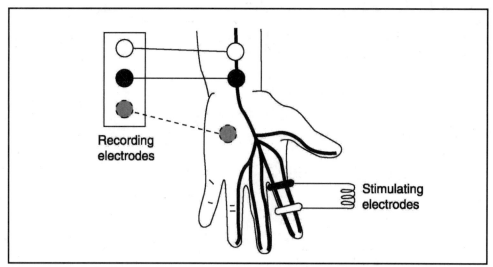

Figure 2-15. Orthodromic method for sensory study of the median nerve.

Objective: *At the conclusion of this laboratory session, the reader will be able to perform tests of the most commonly tested sensory nerves.*

1. Set up for sensory nerve conduction testing:
    A. Set sensitivity at 10 or 20 μV/div
    B. Set sweep at 2 ms/div
    C. Stimulus
        a. Rate—1/sec
        b. Duration—0.05 ms or 0.1 if needed to obtain response
    D. Set filter/frequency responses at 20 Hz to 2 kHz
2. Subject positioning
    A. Supine
    B. Arm fully supported—abducted from side approximately 30 degrees
3. Nerves
    A. Median nerve (Figure 2-15 shows the electrode placement and stimulation site)
        a. Electrode placement—ground is over the dorsum of the hand for both ulnar and median nerve studies

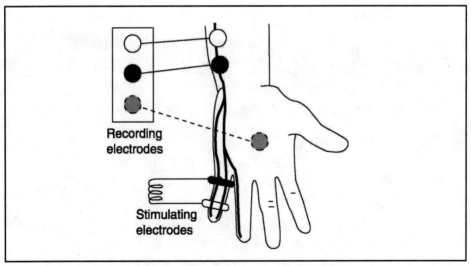

Figure 2-16. Orthodromic method for sensory study of the ulnar nerve.

    i. Orthodromic

       1. Recording electrodes (disc) are placed over the course of the median nerve at the wrist

         A. Recording electrode is distal

         B. Reference is proximal (2.5 to 3 cm from recording electrode); these electrodes must be firmly attached.

       2. Stimulating electrodes—ring electrodes, stimulate second and/or third digits

         A. The negative electrode is proximal and placed over the mid-proximal phalanx

         B. Positive electrode is distal and placed over the middle phalanx at least 2 cm away

    ii. Antidromic

       1. Record with ring electrodes

         A. Recording electrode is proximal (over midproximal phalanx)

         B. Reference electrode is distal over middle phalanx; record from both the second and third digits

       2. Stimulate at the wrist over the course of the median nerve (as in motor nerve studies)

B. Ulnar nerve

   a. Electrode placement

      i. Orthodromic (Figure 2-16 shows the electrode placement and stimulation site)

1. Record with surface electrodes over the course of the ulnar nerve at the wrist
   A. Recording electrode (negative) distal
   B. Reference electrode (positive) is proximal, 2.5 to 3.0 cm from recording electrode
2. Stimulate fifth digit—proximal electrode should be negative, distal electrode is positive placed as described for the median nerve but on the fifth digit

ii. Antidromic
   1. Stimulate at the wrist along the course of the ulnar nerve (as in a motor study)
   2. Record with digital ring electrodes (fifth digit) with the recording (negative) electrode over midproximal phalanx
   3. Reference (positive) electrode over middle phalanx

Measurement of the distance between the stimulating and recording electrodes of the ulnar and median nerves should be done prior to stimulation. This distance should be 12 to 16 cm. Conduction velocities may be calculated on the sensory portion of the ulnar and median nerves by adding additional stimulation sites that are the same as the motor stimulation sites when doing antidromic studies. Conduction velocities can be calculated directly by dividing the distance by the latency since both stimulation and recording are from neural tissue.

C. Sural nerve (antidromic) (Figure 2-17 shows the electrode placement and stimulation site)
   a. Recording electrode
      i. Palpate the nerve behind and below the lateral malleolus and mark, cleanse the skin, and secure the electrode
   b. Reference electrode
      i. Secure the reference electrode distal to and in line with the course of the nerve, 2 to 3 cm from the recording electrode
   c. Ground—medial malleolus
   d. Stimulating electrode
      i. Stimulate over the lateral or posterior surface of the lower leg, 10 to 14 cm proximal to the recording electrode along the lateral border of the lateral gastrocnemius/soleus tendon

D. Radial sensory nerve (superficial radial nerve—antidromic) (Figure 2-18 shows electrode placement and stimulation site)
   a. Recording electrode—placed over the largest palpable branch of the nerve as it crosses the extensor tendon to the thumb or palpate the branch in the anatomical snuff box
   b. Reference electrode—3 to 3.5 cm distal over the dorsum of the first metacarpal

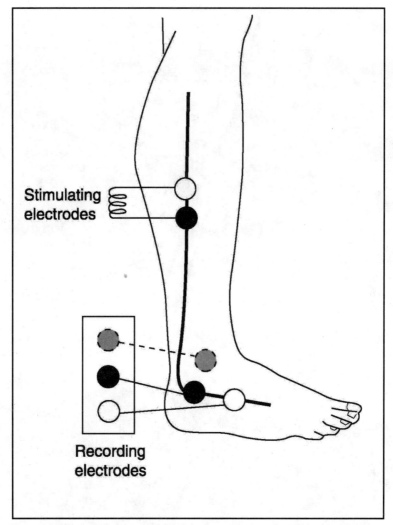

Figure 2-17. Antidromic method for sensory study of the sural nerve.

c. Ground—mid-dorsum of the hand

d. Sites of stimulation

   i. 10 to 14 cm proximal to the recording electrode over the dorsum of the forearm next to the cephalic vein

   ii. Elbow in groove between brachioradialis and brachialis muscle

   iii. Lateral arm—10 cm above lateral epicondyle

e. Alternative radial sensory recording method (antidromic)

   i. Recording electrode—ring electrode over the proximal phalanx of the thumb

   ii. Reference electrode—ring electrode over the distal phalanx of the thumb

   iii. Ground—over dorsum of hand

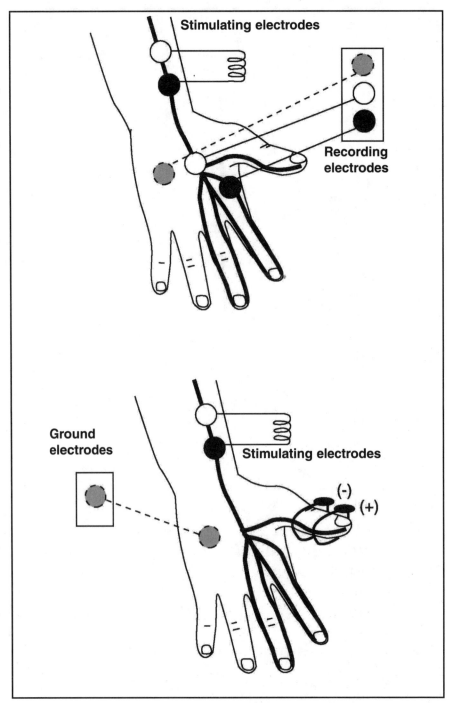

Figure 2-18. Two methods for antidromic radial sensory nerve study.

E. Superficial fibular (peroneal nerve) (sensory) (antidromic)

    a. Recording electrode—anterior ankle just above a line connecting the medial and lateral malleoli—approximately 3 cm medial to the lateral malleolus

    b. Reference electrode 2.5 to 3 cm distal and in line with the recording electrode

    c. Ground electrode—on the lower crest of the tibia between the recording and stimulating electrodes

    d. Stimulation sites—10 to 14 cm from the recording electrode on the anterolateral leg—anterior to the tendon of the peroneus longus muscle

4. Reporting results of the lab exercise (calculating velocities is optional)

  A. Median nerve

    a. Distal latency .... _____ms

    b. Distance .... _____cm

    c. Amplitude .... _____µV

  B. Ulnar nerve

    a. Distal latency .... _____ms

    b. Distance .... _____cm

    c. Amplitude .... _____µV

  C. Sural nerve

    a. Distal latency .... _____ms

    b. Distance .... _____cm

    c. Amplitude .... _____µV

  D. Radial sensory nerve

    a. Distal latency .... _____ms

    b. Distance .... _____cm

    c. Amplitude .... _____µV

  E. Superficial fibular (peroneal) nerve

    a. Distal latency .... _____ms

    b. Distance .... _____cm

    c. Amplitude .... _____µV

5. Normal values

  A. Median nerve

    a. Distal latency: 2.0 to 3.8 ms

    b. Amplitude: 20 to 90 + µV

B. Ulnar nerve
  a. Distal latency: 2.0 to 3.8 ms
  b. Amplitude: 20 to 90 + µV

C. Sural nerve
  a. Conduction velocity: (7 to 21 cm) = 42.55 m/sec
  b. Distal latency: (14 cm) = 3.2 to 4.0 ms
  c. Amplitude: (14 cm) = 20 to 60 µV

D. Radial sensory nerve
  a. Conduction velocity: 60 to 65 m/sec
  b. Distal latency: 1.8 to 2.4 ms
  c. Amplitude: 10 to 35 µV

E. Superficial fibular (peroneal) nerve
  a. Conduction velocity: 51 m/sec
  b. Distal latency: 3.2 to 4.2 ms
  c. Amplitude: 10 to 25 µV

CASE HISTORY 1

Ulnar Nerve

HISTORY

The patient is a 50-year-old male who works as a machinist at a local shipyard. He complains of weakness in his hand and numbness of the fourth and fifth fingers. He does not relate his problem to a specific injury and states onset of symptoms has been gradual over a 10-week period. On questioning, he states he often "bumps" his elbow as part of his job but does not relate this to his symptoms. The patient has worked at his current job for more than 25 years.

PHYSICAL EXAMINATION

The patient has a marked reduction of sensation in response to pin prick over the fifth finger and the ulnar half of the fourth finger. Decreased sensation extends above the wrist on the ulnar side of the forearm. Manual muscle testing shows that the patient has muscle grades of 1/5 in the dorsal interossei, and palmar interossei muscles, 2/5 in the adductor digiti minimi, 3/5 in the ulnar portion of the flexor digitorum profundus, and 3+/5 in the flexor carpi ulnaris. The patient has a positive Tinel's sign at the elbow over the ulnar nerve and a positive elbow flexion test. Phalen's test was negative for the ulnar and median nerves at the wrist.

NERVE CONDUCTION VELOCITY RESULTS

The results of testing the median nerve were normal (Table 2-12). The ulnar nerve showed marked slowing of conduction across the elbow segment, marked decrease in amplitude of the motor response, a 50% decrease in amplitude at the elbow and sites above, and loss of sensory response on sensory conduction testing.

ELECTROMYOGRAPHY RESULTS

- ✦ Abductor pollicis brevis (APB)—Normal (no spontaneous activity, normal motor units on volition, normal recruitment and interference pattern)
- ✦ Flexor carpi radialis (FCR)—Normal (as above)
- ✦ First dorsal interosseus (1st DI)—Fibrillation potentials and sharp waves on needle insertion and probing, no activity was found on attempted muscle contraction
- ✦ Third dorsal interosseus (3rd DI)—Fibrillation potentials and sharp waves on needle insertion and probing
- ✦ Occasional motor unit firing on volition, repetitive firing (single motor unit pattern) on attempted full muscle contraction

Table 2-12 · NCV TEST RESULTS OF CASE 1

Median Nerve

	Latency (ms)	Distance (cm)	Amplitude (mV)	Velocity (m/sec)
Wrist	3.4	8.0	14.0	
Elbow	7.8	23.5	14.0	53
Upper arm	10.1	14.5	13.5	63
Sensory (Second Digit)	3.2	16.0	23.0 µV	
Sensory (Third Digit)	3.2	16.0	23.0 µV	

Ulnar Nerve

Wrist	3.9	8	1.8	
BE	8.6	24	0.9	51
AE	14.8	13	0.9	21
Upper Arm	16.6	16	0.8	56
Sensory (fifth digit)		No response		

✧ Abductor digiti minimi (ADM)—Fibrillation potentials and sharp waves on needle insertion and probing

✧ 1 or 2 motor units on volition, repetitive firing (single motor unit pattern) on attempted full muscle contraction

✧ Flexor digitorum profundus (FDP) (ulnar portion)

✧ Fibrillation potentials on needle insertion

✧ Highly polyphasic motor units, marked decrease in recruitment, interference pattern markedly reduced

✧ Flexor carpi ulnaris (FCU)—No spontaneous activity

✧ Normal motor units and polyphasic potentials

✧ Marked decrease in recruitment, interference pattern reduced (1/2 normal)

DISCUSSION

This patient is an example of extreme nerve compression and damage at the level of the elbow of the ulnar nerve. The loss of a sensory response, slowing of conduction in the segment across the elbow, the decrease in motor amplitudes in general, and the 50% reduction at the elbow sites are all nerve conduction changes indicating the severity and location of the problem. His severity is confirmed by the EMG changes, which indicate severe partial denervation of the muscles supplied by the ulnar nerve.

CASE HISTORY 2

Median Nerve

HISTORY

The patient has a problem of numbness of the fingers (index and middle) and thumb of the right hand, which has been intermittent for approximately 1 year. The patient is a 28-year-old female who works for an insurance broker. Her primary job is data entry using a computer keyboard. She has been working at this job for approximately 6 years. She states that her job has gradually required increased use of the computer over the past 2 years. Prior to this, much of the office work was done other ways. The patient's primary hobby is needlework, which she states has become increasingly difficult for her to do.

PHYSICAL EXAMINATION

The patient has a positive Phalen's test and reverse Phalen's test. The patient complains of increased pain with palpation over the carpal tunnel area. The patient has a positive Tinel's sign over the median nerve at the wrist. Tinel's sign is negative for the ulnar nerve at the wrist and elbow. On sensory testing, the patient has decreased response to pin prick over the volar surface of the index finger and middle finger. Two-point discrimination over the middle finger is 6 mm, 5 mm over the index finger. The left hand by comparison has 2 mm difference in the same area. On manual muscle testing the patient has a 4+/5 abductor pollicis brevis. No atrophy of the thenar eminence is noted.

NERVE CONDUCTION VELOCITY RESULTS

The patient had normal results on testing the ulnar nerve (Table 2-13). The median nerve showed prolonged distal motor and sensory latencies, decreased amplitude of sensory responses, and normal conduction velocities

See Figures 2-19 and 2-20 for waveforms obtained during MNCV testing. Figure 2-19 shows the waveforms with screen settings of 2 mV /div and 2 ms/div. These settings make clear for visual inspection the latency and amplitude of each waveform.

Figure 2-20 shows the same information at 5 mV/div and 5ms/div. Visual inspection of these waveforms shows that the latency and amplitude information is not as easily interpreted.

ELECTROMYOGRAPHY RESULTS

✧   APB—No spontaneous activity, normal motor units, increased polyphasic

Table 2-13

NCV TEST RESULTS OF CASE 2

Median Nerve

Site	Latency (ms)	Distance (cm)	Amplitude (mV)	Velocity (m/sec)
Wrist	4.8*	8.0	8	
Elbow	8.3	21.0	8	60
Upper Arm	10.2	12.0	7.8	63
Sensory (second digit)	3.4*	15.0	19 µV*	
Sensory (third digit)	3.4*	15.0	21 µV*	

Ulnar Nerve

Wrist	3.2	8	11.0	
BE	6.4	20	11.0	63
AE	8.4	12	11.0	60
UA	10.3	12	10.5	63
Sensory (fifth digit)	2.3	15	60.0 µV	

*Indicates abnormal findings

motor units (20%), large motor units up to 8 mV, decreased recruitment of motor units, and decreased interference pattern on volition.

✦ ADM—Normal

✦ 1st DI—Normal

✦ FCR—Normal

✦ Extensor carpi ulnaris (ECU)—Normal

DISCUSSION

The clinical and electromyographic findings of this patient are typical of patients with compression of the median nerve at the wrist. The patient clinically has symptoms and signs of carpal tunnel syndrome. Electromyographic testing showed that the patient had prolonged distal motor and sensory latencies on the median nerve. The patient had decreased amplitude of the sensory potential and EMG changes, indicating chronic neuropathic changes in the thenar eminence.

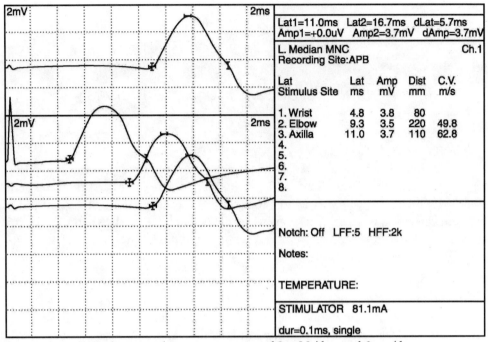

Figure 2-19. Waveforms with screen settings of 2 mV /div and 2 ms/div.

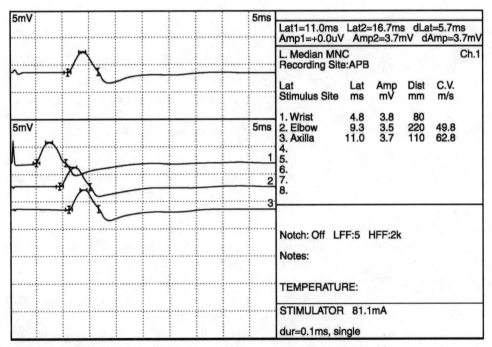

Figure 2-20. Waveforms with screen settings at 5 mV/div and 5ms/div.

CASE HISTORY 3

Fibular (Peroneal) and Tibial Nerves

HISTORY

The patient is a 54-year-old male who works as a member of the crew of a fishing boat. His complaint of numbness of the feet is more severe on the left than the right. The patient has a history of adult-onset diabetes, now treated with insulin. The patient has not always been responsive to medical advice in the treatment of this problem. Current problems have been present for approximately 3 months.

PHYSICAL EXAMINATION

The patient shows atrophic changes in the lower extremities, such as decreased hair growth and dry scaly skin. The feet are cold to touch. The patient has reduced sensation to pin prick below the knees bilaterally. Ankle jerk reflexes are absent, knee jerk reflexes are normal. The patient has decreased response to vibration sense over the tips and base of toes as well as the dorsum of both feet.

NERVE CONDUCTION VELOCITY RESULTS

The fibular nerves bilaterally show slowing of conduction velocities, especially in the distal segment (Table 2-14). Sural sensory responses were absent bilaterally. Tibial nerve conduction velocities were borderline for slowing.

ELECTROMYOGRAPHY RESULTS

The tibialis anterior—No spontaneous activity was noted bilaterally. The patient showed normal motor units mixed with larger than normal motor units (6 mV) and large polyphasic motor units on volition. The patient had poor recruitment of motor units and had a repetitive motor unit interference pattern. Similar findings were obtained in the peroneus longus and extensor digitorum longus muscles bilaterally. The extensor digitorum brevis muscles bilaterally showed sparse fibrillation potentials and positive sharp waves. On voluntary contraction, only very large motor units (8 to 10 mV) were seen in a single motor unit interference pattern. The gastrocnemius muscle bilaterally showed mostly large normal motor units with poor recruitment of smaller motor units and interference patterns that were partially complete (2/3 normal). The abductor hallucis muscle bilaterally showed a few fibrillation potentials on needle insertion and probing. Very little voluntary activity was elicited.

Table 2-14

NCV TEST RESULTS OF CASE 3

Fibular (Peroneal) Nerve

Anatomic Site	Latency (ms)		Distance (cm)		Amplitude (mV)		NCV (m/sec)	
	L	R	L	R	L	R	L	R
Anterior Ankle	4.9	4.4	8.0	8.0	2.0 K	2.2 K		
Below Head	14.2	13.3	30.0	29.5	1.5 K	2.0 K	32	33
Popliteal Space	16.4	15.4	10.0	10.0	1.5 K	2.0 K	45	48
Upper Arm								
Tibial Nerve								
Medial Malleolus	7.7	7.0	14.0	14.0	4.5 K	4.5 K		
Popliteal Space	18.1	16.9	40.5	40.0	4.0 K	4.5 K	39	40

No sural nerve responses could be obtained bilaterally.

DISCUSSION

The fibular (peroneal) NCVs, especially the distal segment from the fibular head to the ankle, were slow and showed less than normal amplitudes. Sural sensory conduction could not be demonstrated. Tibial NCVs were borderline for slowing. The EMG findings were indicative of neuropathic changes of a chronic nature. It can be conjectured that because the patient has diabetes, it is quite likely that all of the above abnormalities are indicative of a peripheral neuropathic process. Diabetes is the likely cause of his current problem, which the electrophysiologic examination does not tell you; therefore, other causes should be ruled out by the referring practitioner. Testing of the upper extremities would be justified in this patient to examine for the effects of neuropathic changes.

CASE HISTORY 4

Table 2-15

NCV RESULTS OF CASE 4

Radial Nerve

Anatomic Site	Latency (ms)		Distance (cm)		Amplitude (mV)		NCV (m/sec)	
	L	R	L	R	L	R	L	R
Forearm	2.8		8.0		6.6 K			
Lateral Arm	5.7		1.7		6.3 K		59	
Supraclavicular or Erb's Point	10.4		31.0		3.0 K		66	

No radial sensory response could be obtained.

Radial Nerve

Case report in a typical reporting format:

Referring diagnosis: Radial nerve compression (Lt)
Testing requested: Examination of Lt upper extremity
Referred by: *Date*:
Problem: Patient has had a wrist drop for 4 weeks

HISTORY

The 29-year-old male patient states that he slept on his arm and awoke with loss of motion in the wrist and finger extensors. No other medical problems are noted in the chart or by the patient.

PHYSICAL EXAMINATION

Manual muscle test reveals 0/5 activity in the thumb extensor, finger extensors, wrist extensors, and brachioradialis. Triceps tested at 4/5. All other upper extremity muscles tested at 5/5 (normal).

NERVE CONDUCTION VELOCITY RESULTS

Nerve conduction velocity of the radial nerve is normal (Table 2-15); however, there is a significant drop in amplitude at the supraclavicular site of stimulation compared to the lower sites.

MNCV tests of ulnar and median nerves were within normal limits.

Electromyography Results

Extensor pollicis longus—No spontaneous activity; no activity or attempted volition.

Extensor carpi radialis longus—No spontaneous activity; on volition, only one or two motor units were seen.

Brachioradialis—No spontaneous activity; on volition, few motor units were seen; interference pattern was a single motor unit pattern.

Lateral head of triceps—Revealed no spontaneous activity and normal motor units on volition and normal recruitment and interference pattern. The abductor digiti minimi, flexor carpi ulnaris, abductor pollicis brevis, and flexor carpi radialis all tested as normal.

Assessment

The patient is demonstrating a conduction block (partial neuropraxia) of the radial nerve in the area above the superficial radial nerve branch and below the innervation of the triceps. No spontaneous activity was found, and the patient's conduction on the radial nerve is retained. There is a significant drop in amplitude at the supraclavicular site compared to the lateral arm site of stimulation that also helps to localize the area of compression. Today's findings are good prognostic indicators for recovery of function within 3 months of the onset of his problems. If the expected recovery does not take place, retesting would be indicated.

Review Questions

1. Describe the characteristics that may be measured when a conduction study is performed. What is the importance of each characteristic?

2. Describe the process for computing a nerve conduction velocity.

3. Explain the difference between orthodromic and antidromic stimulation of sensory nerves.

4. Outline the general procedures for performing a conduction velocity test.

5. List the sites of stimulation for performing a motor nerve conduction test of the (a) fibular (peroneal) nerve, (b) median nerve, and (c) femoral nerve.

6. Describe the settings on the EMG machine for motor conduction testing and sensory conduction testing. Explain the differences.

7. When testing the ulnar and median nerves in the upper arm area, what factors should one watch for and what could be the cause of the problem(s)?

Electromyography

OBJECTIVES

At the end of this unit of study the reader will be able to:

✧ Describe the characteristics of a normal motor unit and elaborate on the expected characteristics of a normal EMG examination.

✧ Describe the characteristics of potentials that occur spontaneously and define the circumstances under which they might occur.

✧ Describe the characteristics of abnormal potentials that occur on volition and define the circumstances under which they might occur.

✧ Perform a clinical EMG examination in a laboratory environment with a normal individual and demonstrate the technique of needle insertion and exploration of normal muscle.

✧ Demonstrate the ability to perform the EMG needle insertion and examination techniques of selected upper and lower extremity muscles.

✧ Recognize the appearance of normal and abnormal findings by sight on the screen (oscilloscope) and by sound on the loudspeaker of the various normal and abnormal EMG potentials.

✧ Perform, with the guidance of an experienced clinical examiner, a clinical EMG examination.

Table 3-1

CHARACTERISTICS OF NORMAL MOTOR UNITS

Voltage (Amplitude)
100 µV to 4000 to 5000 µV (4 to 5 mV)

Duration
2 to 17 ms, most are 8 to 12 ms

Waveform
Mono to four phase, most are bi- or triphasic; more than four is polyphasic

Frequency
1 to 60/sec, highly variable depending on individual muscles

Sound
Clear, sharp, thump, or plunk. Duration and proximity to needle electrode determine sharpness of sound (Figure 3-1)

Normal Motor Units

GENERAL COMMENTS

The list of characteristics (Table 3-1) is a general guide to the important data about the normal motor unit. Because electromyography is based on lower motor neuron function, the normal motor unit becomes the single most important determinant of normality in electromyography. If the motor unit is not functioning properly, or not functioning at all because of a loss of nerve supply, certain changes will take place that indicate that this is so. Each individual motor unit, as it is displayed on the screen, has characteristics that are unique unto itself regarding the characteristics that are shown above. This means that if a patient is contracting minimally you can recognize different motor units as they are displayed on the screen. As you increase the level of contraction, the patient recruits more and more motor units. On a full contraction, the patient recruits so many motor units that they are firing one after the other and there is no longer any way to distinguish individual motor units. This is known as a *full interference pattern*. This is an important aspect of normal electromyography.

There are characteristic differences in the motor units from one group of muscles to another. Facial muscles tend to be of shorter duration and lower amplitude than skeletal muscles. Extensor muscles tend to be of shorter duration than flexor muscles. Motor unit territory is also important in determining the amplitude. In the intrinsic muscles of the hand, motor unit territories are grouped so that the muscle fibers for individual motor units are relatively close together.

Even though the number of fibers making up the motor unit is not large, poten-

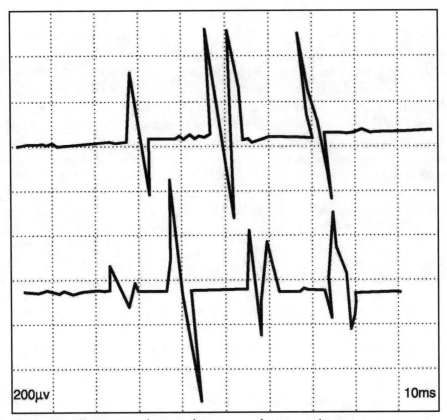

Figure 3-1. Illustration of a waveform, normal motor units.

tials tend to be of larger amplitude than the amplitude of potentials from muscles in which the motor unit territory is widely dispersed, such as in the gastrocnemius. The gastrocnemius muscle motor units often contain up to 2000 fibers but, because of their distribution, do not elicit characteristically large amplitude potentials. As individuals age, the average duration of motor units tends to increase.

The Electromyographic Examination

One of the most important aspects of the EMG examination is a thorough knowledge of the patient's history and clinical findings. It is essential that the EMG examiner examines the patient for clinical details. This means that it is not enough just to read the patient's chart and find another person's description of the patient's abnormalities. For example, it is important for the examiner to know whether the patient has muscle weakness and to have a clinical estimate of this weakness. The examiner should know something about the reflex activity of the patient and other clinical details. It is incumbent upon physical therapists performing EMG examinations to perform thorough clinical examinations of the patient prior to carrying out the electromyographic examination.

The patient should be positioned comfortably so that the muscles to be tested are well exposed and in a position where the patient is relaxed. The ground electrode should be secured to the patient in an appropriate place and the area where the needle electrode is to be inserted should be prepared by cleansing the skin with alcohol. It is important that the insertion of the needle electrode be done so that it causes minimal discomfort. At each insertion site, the patient is observed as the needle is inserted for the type of activity generated by insertion and movement of the needle. Secondly, spontaneous activity should be observed for because in a normal EMG there is electrical silence (ie, no electrical activity displayed) when no active contraction of muscle is taking place. Thirdly, at each needle site the potentials seen on mild, moderate, and maximal contractions should be observed. On voluntary contraction the characteristics described for normal motor units should be observed. It is essential that an adequate number of motor units be analyzed to ensure validity of the test. At each insertion site the *quadrant method* of examining, or the *around the clock method*, should be used. This means that for each insertion site through the skin the muscle is sampled in several areas at varying depths (Figure 3-2). The electromyographer should examine as many needle sites in an individual muscle as he or she feels are necessary to ensure reliability and validity of the examination.

Normal EMG should demonstrate the following:

1. Upon needle insertion, as the needle is moved sharply into the muscle, a brief burst of electrical activity is produced which lasts for 0.5 to 2 seconds and is generally of indistinguishable short duration activity up to 200 µV in size. Some have likened the sound produced by this to the scratch of a needle on a phonograph record. As the needle penetrates into the muscle fibers, the muscle is mechanically stimulated or injured, which gives rise to a short burst of activity.

2. When the muscle is relaxed, no electrical activity should occur in normal individuals.

3. Upon normal contraction, individual motor units should be distinguishable on the screen. These can be examined for the characteristics described for normal motor units. As the strength of contraction is increased, a normal recruitment of more and more motor units occurs. Finally, upon full contraction, a complete interference pattern is obtained, obliterating the ability to evaluate individual motor units because of disruption of the baseline by the amount of activity on the screen. This activity is summated and the amplitude of the interference pattern is larger than the amplitude of individual motor units. Care must be taken to understand the factors that may lead to a less than normal interference pattern in normal individuals. One of these is pain from the needle electrode. Sometimes moving the electrode just a very small amount will allow the patient to achieve a normal interference pattern.

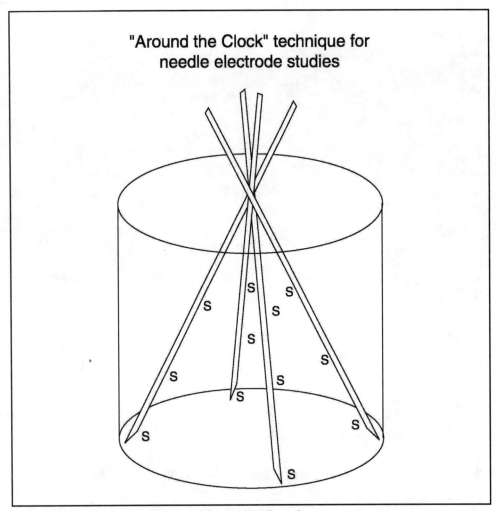

"Around the Clock" technique for needle electrode studies

Figure 3-2. Needle technique for a clinical EMG study.

Spontaneous Potentials

FIBRILLATION POTENTIALS

The origin of *fibrillation potentials* has been assumed to be the muscle fiber. Apparently, this characteristic may be inherent to muscle tissue. Muscle tissue that does not have a nerve supply will tend to fibrillate. This has been demonstrated experimentally by growing muscle from an embryo that has never had a nerve supply. When tested in a laboratory situation, fibrillation potentials occurred. It has been conjectured that the anterior horn cell exerts an influence over muscle fiber, which inhibits fibrillation. Anything that tends to disrupt this process permits the muscle fiber to fibrillate. Changes in the influence of upper motor neurons on the

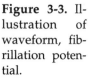

FIBRILLATION POTENTIALS

Table 3-2

Voltage
10 to 300 μV (50 to 100 μV common)

Duration
Usually less than 2 m/sec

Waveform
Biphasic, initial phase positive (+)

Frequency
2 to 30/sec (10 common)

Sound
Sharp, high-pitched click (like rain on a tin roof)

Figure 3-3. Illustration of waveform, fibrillation potential.

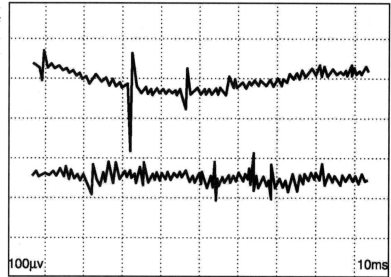

100μv   10ms

anterior horn cells may also permit fibrillation potentials to occur. Some studies have documented this occurrence in patients who have had spinal cord injuries or cerebrovascular accidents and, during a certain critical time period after this, while the anterior horn cell is in a state of disequilibrium, there are fibrillation potentials occurring in muscles whose anterior horn cells are involved. Fibrillation potentials have been considered to be one of the primary indicators of denervation of skeletal muscle and, as such, is a very important EMG finding. It is essential to remember that these potentials are spontaneous (Table 3-2 and Figure 3-3).

Table 3-3

POSITIVE SHARP WAVES

Voltage
50 to 2000 μV (average 100 to 300 μV)

Duration
2 to 1000 ms (average 7 to 10 m/sec)

Waveform
Initial sharp plus deflection with slower negative rise to overlap of baseline

Frequency
2 to 100/sec (10/sec common)

Sound
Sharp click to thud depending on size and duration of waveform

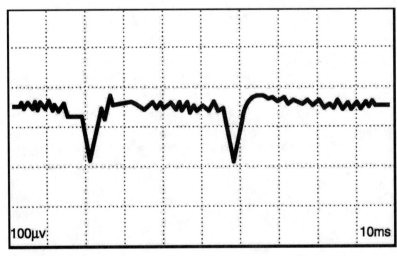

100μv: 10ms

Figure 3-4. Illustration of waveform, positive sharp waves.

POSITIVE SHARP WAVES

Positive sharp waves occur spontaneously. They often occur with fibrillation potentials. The origin of positive sharp waves has not been determined. Some authorities feel that they come from the sarcolemma of muscle. Others feel that they are a single fiber phenomenon, especially a damaged area from a single fiber. A third theory involves multiple fiber discharge. Positive sharp waves are not as common as fibrillation potentials in denervated muscle. They are considered to have the same significance; that is, they are an indication that the muscle has lost its nerve supply (Table 3-3 and Figure 3-4).

MOTOR END-PLATE POTENTIALS

Motor end-plate potentials are found in normal individuals if the needle electrode is placed in the motor end-plate area. It is usually accompanied by pain. Moving the

MOTOR END-PLATE POTENTIALS

Voltage
10 to 300 µV (100 µV common)

Duration
Less than 2 m/sec

Waveform
Biphasic, initial phase negative

Frequency
2 to 30/sec

Sound
Sharp, high-pitched

needle slightly will not only reduce the pain but will also eliminate the motor end-plate potentials. The important distinguishing characteristic between motor end-plate potentials and fibrillation potentials is the direction of the initial biphasic wave that is negative in motor end-plate potentials. In the facial muscle, the motor end-plate area is larger than in skeletal muscle, and it is easier to inadvertently have the needle in the end-plate area when examining facial muscles. Some authors have also described a phenomenon that accompanies end-plate potentials. It is a non-propogated potential considered to correspond to miniature end-plate potentials. These potentials have a high frequency and irregular pattern of discharge with amplitudes, usually of 10 to 40 µV. They have a duration of less than 2 ms, are monophasic, and are negative in direction (Table 3-4 and Figure 3-5).

FASCICULATION POTENTIALS

Fasciculation potentials are motor unit potentials that occur spontaneously. They can be either normal motor unit shape or polyphasic in shape. If they are polyphasic, they have four or more phases. The potentials are often associated with chronic peripheral nerve or nerve root lesions. They are also associated with anterior horn cell disease, especially irritative lesions of the anterior horn cell, and have been associated with such diseases as amyotrophic lateral sclerosis and progressive spinal muscular atrophy (PSMA). In these conditions, the fasciculation potentials must be found widespread throughout the body, not just in one or two sites or only one extremity (Table 3-5 and Figure 3-6).

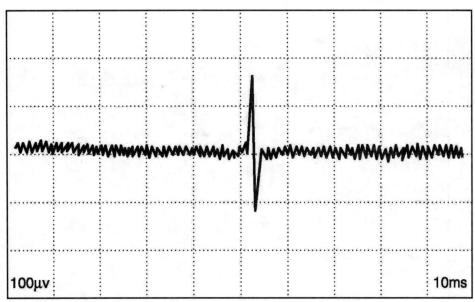

Figure 3-5. Illustration of waveform, motor end-plate potentials.

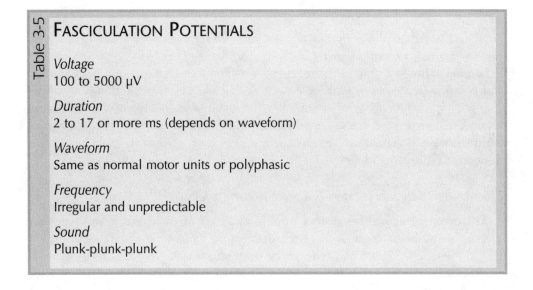

Table 3-5

FASCICULATION POTENTIALS

Voltage
100 to 5000 µV

Duration
2 to 17 or more ms (depends on waveform)

Waveform
Same as normal motor units or polyphasic

Frequency
Irregular and unpredictable

Sound
Plunk-plunk-plunk

Volitional Potentials

POLYPHASIC POTENTIALS

These potentials are among the most important in clinical EMG. *Polyphasic potentials* may be indicative of degenerating lesions, regenerating lesions, and chronic compressive lesions of peripheral motor axons. Polyphasic potentials in small

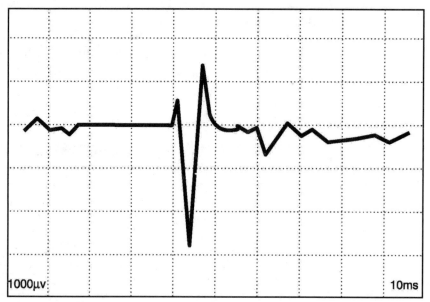

Figure 3-6. Illustration of waveform, fasciculation potential.

numbers (less than 10% of potentials seen) may be seen in normal individuals. Very small polyphasic potentials are typically of short duration and low amplitude and are indicative of the first signs of the regeneration of peripheral nerve lesions. There are also polyphasic potentials that have been described as "short-duration, low-amplitude polyphasic potentials" that are indicative of an acute neuropathic or myopathic process. Larger polyphasic potentials are indicative of chronicity in the neuropathic process. Polyphasic potentials are found in both myopathic and neuropathic disorders (Table 3-6 and Figure 3-7).

GIANT OR LARGER THAN NORMAL MOTOR UNIT POTENTIALS

The designation *giant motor unit* is no longer used by many electromyographers. These potentials are referred to as *larger than normal motor units* when describing the motor units seen. These potentials can be similar to normal motor units in shape or polyphasic in shape. The most important characteristic of these potentials is their enormous amplitude. They indicate a chronicity of the neuropathic lesion, and they are primarily based on the phenomenon of axonal branching or imperfect renervation following complete nerve lesion that alters the motor unit territory. Larger than normal motor unit potentials are often found accompanying other abnormal potentials, particularly polyphasic potentials (Table 3-7 and Figure 3-8).

ABNORMAL MOTOR UNIT POTENTIALS

Most authors do not acknowledge these potentials when discussing electromyography. These are potentials that do occur and are very similar to normal motor

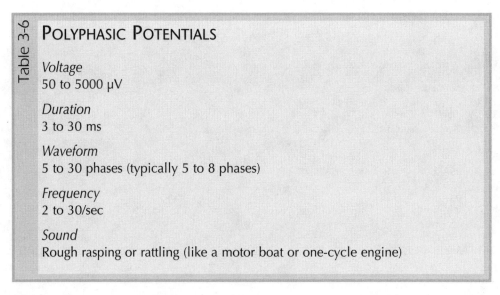

Table 3-6

POLYPHASIC POTENTIALS

Voltage
50 to 5000 μV

Duration
3 to 30 ms

Waveform
5 to 30 phases (typically 5 to 8 phases)

Frequency
2 to 30/sec

Sound
Rough rasping or rattling (like a motor boat or one-cycle engine)

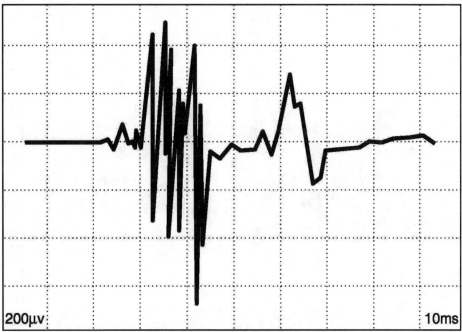

200μv   10ms

Figure 3-7. Illustration of waveform, polyphasic potential.

unit potentials but are either shorter or longer in duration. They may occur accompanying polyphasic potentials and are found more frequently in some individuals than in others. They are mentioned here for the sake of completeness and to make the reader aware that these potentials may occur. (I consider them to have the same significance as polyphasic potentials. One axiom of electromyography is that if you do not understand a potential you just do not describe it. I think that it is time

Table 3-7

LARGER THAN NORMAL ("GIANT") MOTOR UNITS

Voltage
Greater than 5000 µV (5 mV to 25 mV)

Duration
4 to 5 msec to 25 to 30 msec

Waveform
NMU to polyphasic waveforms

Frequency
Same as NMU and polyphasic potentials

Sound
Varies from thump to polyphasic sounds (Figure 3-8)

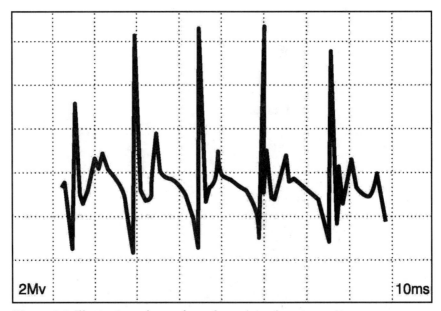

2Mv   10ms

Figure 3-8. Illustration of waveform, large (giant) motor units.

examiners started acknowledging these potentials and mentioning the fact that they are being seen.) (Table 3-8 and Figure 3-9)

MYOPATHIC POTENTIALS

Many electromyographers have dropped the designation of *myopathic potentials*. These potentials are of short duration. The reason for retaining them as a separate category is to highlight the myopathic origin of these very short-duration, low-

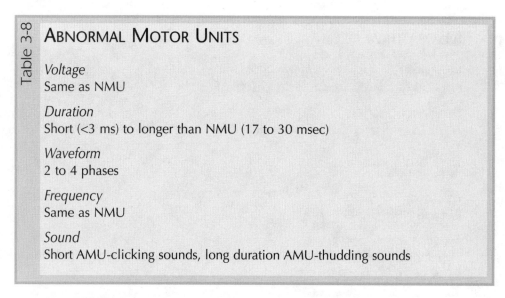

Table 3-8

ABNORMAL MOTOR UNITS

Voltage
Same as NMU

Duration
Short (<3 ms) to longer than NMU (17 to 30 msec)

Waveform
2 to 4 phases

Frequency
Same as NMU

Sound
Short AMU-clicking sounds, long duration AMU-thudding sounds

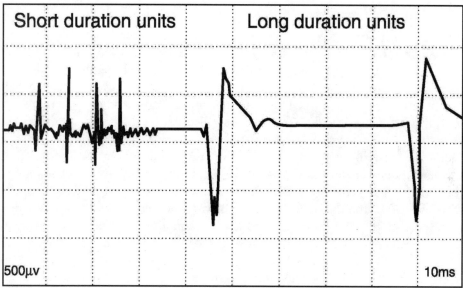

Figure 3-9. Illustration of waveform, abnormal motor units.

amplitude potentials. Myopathic potentials are potentials that indicate primary muscle disease and, as such, are different than the neuropathic potentials we have described. These myopathic potentials are decreased in size and duration when compared to normal motor units. In severe myopathic changes, the waveform can be so shortened and diminished in amplitude that the potentials resemble fibrillation potentials, except that they occur upon volition.

When discussing myopathic potentials it must be understood that we are not discussing all the EMG abnormalities that occur in the myopathic process. Over time

Table 3-9

Myopathic Potentials

Voltage
Generally lower, decreased to 50 to 300 µV

Duration
Average duration of motor unit shortened (can be very short, 2 to 3 ms)

Waveform
Same as NMU

Frequency
Same as NMU

Sound
Higher pitch due to decreased duration; clicks, can resemble sounds of fibrillation potentials when severe

it has generally been accepted that during the myopathic process, fibrillation potentials and positive sharp waves may be found. This may be the result of the myopathic process involving the distal portion of the axon and the motor end-plate. It also has been noted that on volition, in addition to myopathic potentials, polyphasic potentials may also occur. This is an indication of the changes within the motor unit. In most myopathic disorders there is a distribution that is characteristic, especially in the early stages, of the myopathy for that particular myopathic disease. An example is the limb girdle changes found in muscular dystrophy. This means that in the same individual, myopathic potentials can be found in some muscles along with the accompanying changes, and in other muscles the patient will be absolutely normal. Therefore, the distribution of myopathic findings is important. The reason these potentials are of short duration and low amplitude is that as the myopathic process becomes evident, individual muscle fibers no longer function effectively and drop out of the motor unit. As this process progresses, fewer functioning muscle fibers are available in that individual motor unit. Also, as a result of the myopathic process, a moderate contraction will result in a full interference pattern (Table 3-9 and Figure 3-10).

Myotonic Potentials and Complex Repetitive Discharges

Myotonic discharges are found in diseases in which myotonia is a prominent feature, such as congenital myotonia. These potential sounds are so characteristic that they have been described by some people as the only truly characteristic diagnostic potential in EMG. This statement is misleading because myotonic potentials may occur in individuals who have conditions other than myotonia.

The term *complex repetitive discharge* has come to mean any recurring action potentials with the same or nearly the same form. These potentials have been called a variety of names (bizarre high-frequency potentials, pseudomyotonic potentials).

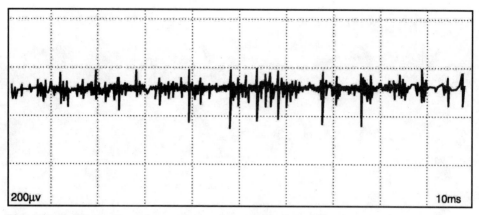

200μv   10ms

Figure 3-10. Illustration of waveform, myopathic potentials.

These potentials can occur during contraction or while the muscle is at rest. These potentials have been found in normal individuals and in individuals with chronic nerve root and peripheral nerve deficits. The major difference between these and myotonic potentials is that these potentials fire at a regular rate and do not decrease and increase in frequency or amplitude as do myotonic potentials. This means that this sound is more characteristically like a machine gun than like a dive bomber. Complex repetitive discharges do not have a specific diagnostic significance but often occur in long-standing disorders or occasionally in normal individuals without explanation (Tables 3-10 and 3-11, and Figure 3-11).

ARTIFACTS

Artifacts have been described as potentials or signals that are not generated by the process under evaluation. These potentials do not arise from the muscle in which the needle electrode is inserted. A common artifact is a cardiac potential, especially when doing the facial muscles and chest muscles. These should be readily recognized because of the regular occurrence and characteristic waveform.

Change the settings on your oscilloscope to display the complete waveform, which should resemble an electrocardiogram. Diathermy causes interference with the waveform, making it impossible to see EMG potentials. Defective needle insulation of monopolar needles and defects in the protective insulation between the reference and recording electrodes of a coaxial needle are often the source of an artifact. These conditions form a short circuit, and the potentials displayed are often bizarre-looking potentials. Improper grounding will often permit AC interference or other disturbances in the shape of the baseline. Whenever potentials are displayed that you feel are not associated with the muscle under evaluation, an attempt should be made to discover the source. This will help you to eliminate that particular artifact. Patients who have tremors often display tremor activity during an EMG evaluation. *Tremor potentials* are small bursts of regular, normal-appearing motor units that occur at regular intervals, and tremor counts can be done. Subclinical Parkinson's disease often displays this phenomenon. Some people have said that

MYOTONIC DISCHARGE

Voltage
Increases and decreases—small up to 3000 µV (steady in bizarre high-frequency discharges)

Duration
Depends on frequency (5 to 20 ms)

Waveform
Regular (repeats) some are biphasic, some are positive phases only

Frequency
20 to 60/sec (varies)

Sound
Like a dive bomber as voltage increases and decreases

REPETITIVE DISCHARGE

Voltage
Up to 3000 µV (does not vary significantly)

Duration
5 to 20 ms

Waveform
Regular and repetitive (does not change)

Frequency
20 to 50/sec

Sound
High-pitched, repetitive sound (like a machine gun)

these parkinsonian tremor potential sounds are like that of a train "chugging" down the track. These are not artifacts but are unexpected findings in some patients, and understanding this may avoid confusion.

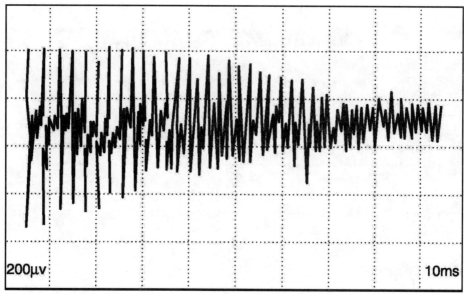

Figure 3-11. Illustration of waveform, myotonic potentials.

Bibliography

Aminoff MJ. General aspects of needle electromyography. Clinical aspects of needle electromyography. In: Aminoff MJ, ed. *Electromyography in Clinical Practice*. 3rd ed. NY: Churchill Livingstone, 1998: 63-85, 87-112.

Dimitru D. Needle electromyography. In: Dimitru D, ed. *Electrodiagnostic Medicine*. Philadelphia, Pa: Hanley and Belfus; 1995: 211-245.

Eddy JG, Snyder-Mackler L. Clinical electrophysiologic testing. In: Robinson A, Snyder-Mackler L, eds. *Clinical Electrophysiology*. 2nd ed. Baltimore, Md: Williams and Wilkins; 1998.

Geiringer SR. *Anatomic Localization for Needle Electromyograph*. 2nd ed. Philadelphia, Pa: Hanley and Belfus; 1999.

Goodgold J. *Anatomical Correlates of Clinical Electromyography*. 2nd ed. Baltimore, Md: Williams and Wilkins; 1984.

Johnson EW, Pease WS, eds. *Practical Electromyography*. 2nd ed. Baltimore, Md: Williams and Wilkins; 1997.

Liveson JA. Interpretation of electrodiagnostic data. In: Liveson JA, ed. *Peripheral Neurology: Case Studies in Electrodiagnosis*. 2nd ed. Philadelphia, Pa: FA Davis; 1991.

Nestor D, Nelson RM. Electrophysiologic evaluation: an overview. In: Nelson RM, Hayes KW, Currier DP, eds. *Clinical Electrotherapy*. 2nd ed. Baltimore, Md: Williams and Wilkins; 1999: chap 12.

Perotto A. *Anatomic Guide for the Electromyographer*. 3rd ed. Springfield, Ill: Charles C. Thomas; 1994.

Stahlberg E. Needle electromyography. In: Johnson EW, Pease WS, eds. *Practical Electromyography*. 3rd ed. Baltimore, Md: Williams and Wilkins; 1997: 89-113.

LABORATORY EXERCISE 6
Clinical EMG Techniques

Table 3-12

TYPICAL SETTINGS FOR NEEDLE EMG

Setting	At Rest	Minimal Contraction	Maximal Contraction
Sweep speed	10	10	10 to 100 (time/div) ms
Sensitivity	50/100	100-500	500 to 2000 (mV/div)
Filter	—	20 Hz to 10 kHz	—
Audio	On	On	On

OBJECTIVE

At the completion of this laboratory exercise the reader should be able to safely insert a needle electrode in muscle and explore the parameters of normal potentials. (If you have any objections to being a subject during this laboratory session please notify an instructor.)

1. Instrumentation and supplies—During this lab, universal precautions should be observed (see Appendix C)

   A. Assemble:

      a. Needle electrodes (disposable electrodes)

      b. Alcohol, swabs, surface electrode, ground

      c. Electrode, gel, protective gloves

   B. Set up the unit in EMG mode (Table 3-12).

   C. After examining your subject and agreeing on a muscle for sampling (arms and legs only), place the subject on the table with the extremity to be examined adequately supported.

   D. Do all the palpating that you wish to do, then clean the area with an alcohol swab. Let the alcohol dry.

   E. Place the ground and reference electrode if using a monopolar needle.

   F. Remove a sterile needle electrode from the disposable pack and insert it. (Never use a needle that has touched a nonsterile surface, or one that has been used before.)

2. Recording of potentials (Table 3-13)

   A. With the needle ready to be inserted in the muscle and after it is inserted, observe:

Table 3-13	RECORDING OF POTENTIALS			
	Record	1st Potential	2nd Potential	3rd Potential
	Amplitude			
	Duration			
	Waveform			
	Frequency			
	Sound			

     a. Insertional noise (by advancing the electrode)

     b. Spontaneous activity—if present

     c. Single motor unit potentials

     d. Minimal contraction gradually advancing to maximal contraction

     e. Resting activity—observe for 1 minute following maximal contraction

     f. Single motor unit potentials. Move the needle so that it is near a motor unit.

  B. Repeat this for at least two other motor units by moving the needle to another site. The subjects should not experience continuous pain. If they have pain, reposition the electrode immediately or remove the electrode and ask for assistance.

3. Continuation of recording potentials

  A. Move the needle electrode to the extensor muscles of the forearm.

  B. Observe the muscle you select at rest, during slight contraction, and on maximal contraction. Record your observation in the same manner as above. (If you observe any unusual potentials, share them with an instructor.)

  C. Continue the examination by moving near an active motor unit. While the subject maintains his effort, move the needle out of the motor unit territory by withdrawing it slowly.

  D. Move the electrode to a new level. Become aware of differences in tissue resistance as you pass through different layers.

  E. In order to differentiate "near" and "far" EMG activity, have the subject relax the extensor while he contracts only the triceps, only the biceps, only the opponens pollicis, and only the finger flexors.

4. Other muscles

  A. If time permits, examine one of the following:

     a. The opposite extensor at the same site. Do the potentials look the same?

   b. The gastrocnemius on the same side. Do the potentials look the same?

   c. Load the extended fingers or wrist with a book and observe the inter-
       ference pattern as fatigue develops.

B. Have the subject isolate a single motor unit and train it to contract in
    sets—once, twice, etc. Turn down the audio and see if your subject can
    still fire this unit. Block his vision of the screen and ask him to repeat his
    motor unit pattern. Can he do it? When the laboratory session is com-
    plete, dispose of the used needle electrode in a "safe" container that meets
    the standards for disposal of contaminated materials. The laboratory
    instructor should inform you of the rules for the installation where the lab-
    oratory session is taking place.

LABORATORY EXERCISE 7
Clinical EMG Techniques

OBJECTIVE

The reader will identify differences in potentials visually (displayed on the screen) and audibly, and will be able to identify differing characteristics of normal and abnormal potentials.

Procedure

Watch and listen to normal and abnormal EMG potentials. Record observations on this sheet, as noted below.

Diagram the following abnormal potentials noting their duration, amplitude, shape and other special features (eg, initial phase negative or positive—association with pain):

1. Fibrillation potential

2. Positive sharp wave

3. Motor end-plate potentials

4. Fasciculation potential

5. Short-duration, low-amplitude polyphasic potential (SLAP)

6. Long-duration, high-amplitude polyphasic potential

7. Other potentials (myotonic discharge, abnormal motor units, complex repetitive discharges)

Briefly identify the physiological basis for:

1. Normal motor unit potential

2. SLAP

3. Long-duration, high-amplitude polyphasic potential

LABORATORY EXERCISE 8
Lower Extremity EMG Techniques

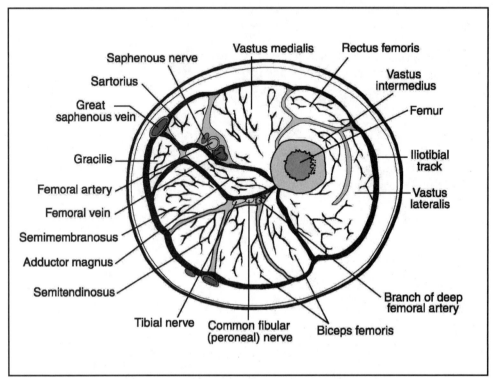

Figure 3-12. Cross section of the lower extremity at mid-thigh.

OBJECTIVES

By the end of this laboratory session the reader will (Figures 3-12 and 3-13):

✧ Develop basic skills in needle electrode EMG techniques in the lower extremity

✧ Perform and record the EMG exam of at least five lower extremity muscles (and observe at least five more)

✧ Practice the technique of achieving isolated contraction of the muscles tested for kinesiological verification of electrode position

Procedures:

1. Equipment

    A. Select EMG mode (see Table 3-12)

    B. Sweep speed—10 ms/div

    C. Sensitivity—50 or 100 mV/div

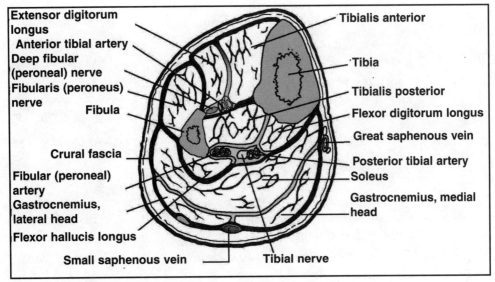

Figure 3-13. Cross section of the lower extremity at mid-calf.

    D. Set equipment so that storage can be achieved if needed.

    E. Turn the speaker volume so that potentials can be heard; remember, you can adjust the volume at any time.

2. Patient

    A. Supine position on the table

    B. Expose only the part of the body you are actually testing at that time; some EMG potentials are altered by cool temperatures, especially in the lower extremities.

    C. You will be testing the following list of muscles:

First Group	**Second Group**
Vastus medialis	Tibialis anterior
Gastrocnemius, lateral head	Extensor digitorum brevis
Fibularis (peroneus) longus	Tensor fasciae latae
Tibialis posterior	Adductor longus/sartorius
Extensor digitorum longus	Abductor hallucis

Additional Muscles (if laboratory time permits)	
Extensor hallucis longus	Abductor digiti minimi
Soleus	Gluteus medius
Biceps femoris	Gluteus maximus

    D. If you are using a monopolar electrode, place the reference electrode over the area adjacent to where you plan to insert the needle. Place the ground electrode on a bony area.

    E. With an alcohol swab, generously wipe all of the areas you plan to test.

3. Pre-Exam Method
   A. Locate the muscle by palpation (using an anatomical reference if needed).
   B. Ask the patient to contract the muscle while you palpate, verifying the location of the muscle.
   C. Teach the patient to isolate the muscle by reducing incidental motions, and by requesting decreasing muscular effort.
   D. Teach the patient minimal contraction effort. (Do not insert the needle until you are successful. If the patient cannot achieve minimal isolated contraction of this muscle, start somewhere else.)

4. Exam Method
   A. Ask the patient to contract the muscle, re-identify the muscle by palpation, and locate the point you plan to insert the electrode. Straddle the point with two fingers of your hand.
   B. Tell the patient to relax—wait until he or she does—then press down with the fingers and spread the skin (tighten). Touch the skin with the needle (hold at a 45-degree angle). Turn on the patient input of the preamplifier. From this point, the sound is important and should be on. Press through the skin with a quick, short thrust. Penetrate the skin quickly.
   C. Use the sound as a guide to where you are and what the patient's status is (eg, relaxed-quiet or tense-noisy).
   D. Achieve silence (patient relaxed, no contractions). As you advance the needle, listen for normal insertion activity. Use short, quick thrusts to advance the needle.
   E. Ask the patient to contract easily. Listen and look at the units. If they are "close" units, verify your location by asking the patient to make isolated, easy contractions of the muscle you are seeking and its nearby neighbors (eg, for vastus medialis the hamstrings, adductors, and sartorius). Do not allow strong contractions or co-contractions when you are attempting to isolate a muscle.
   F. When you have proven your location, begin collecting the following data. Do it in your head while you are performing the test of that muscle. Write it down after you have removed the needle.
      a. Insertion activity
      b. Spontaneous activity (patient at rest)
      c. Motor unit configuration (all factors of importance)
      d. Motor unit recruitment (interference pattern)
   G. Remove the needle.
   H. Move on to the next muscle and repeat the above.
   I. Follow laboratory procedures for disposal of needle electrodes at the completion of the session.

LABORATORY EXERCISE 9
Upper Extremity EMG Techniques

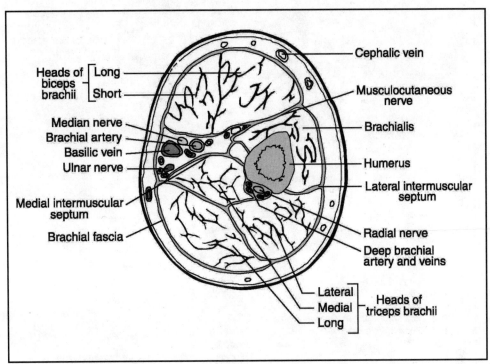

Figure 3-14. Cross section of upper extremity at just below mid-arm.

OBJECTIVES

At the completion of this laboratory session the reader will be able to (Figures 2-9, 3-14, and 3-15):

1. Perform and record the EMG exam of at least six upper extremity muscles (and observe six more).

2. Develop further kinesiological isolation techniques, including use of synergistic patterns.

3. Plan the structure and organization of the EMG exam.

Procedure

A. Equipment (same settings as Lab Exercise 6 [see Table 3-12])

1. EMG mode

2. Sweep speed—10 ms/div

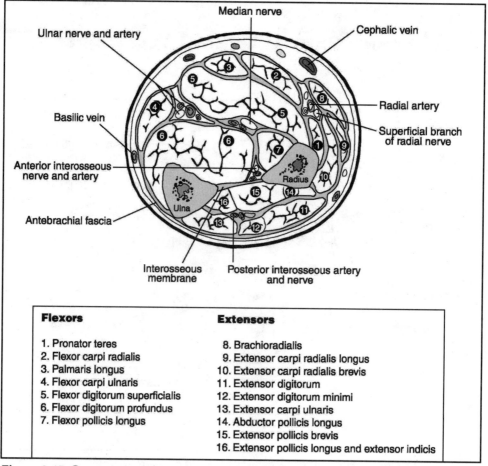

Figure 3-15. Cross section of upper extremity at mid-forearm.

3. Sensitivity—50 or 100 µV/div (set equipment so that storage can be achieved if needed).

4. Prepare for switch to storage mode.

5. Turn the speaker volume so that potentials can be heard.

B. Patient

1. Supine position with upper extremity well supported

2. You will be testing from the following list of muscles:

First Group	Second Group
Deltoid, middle	Triceps, lateral head
Brachioradialis	Flexor carpi ulnaris
Abductor pollicis longus	Flexor digitorum superficialis
Flexor pollicis longus	First dorsal interosseous
Abductor digiti minimi	Abductor pollicis brevis

Additional Muscles—Optional

Biceps   Extensor digitorum communis
Brachialis   Extensor indicis
Extensor pollicis longus   Flexor carpi radialis

3. If you are using a monopolar electrode, place the reference electrode over the area adjacent to where you plan to insert the needle. Place the ground electrode on a bony area.

4. With an alcohol swab, generously wipe all of the areas you plan to test.

C. Pre-Exam Method

1. Locate the muscle by palpation (using an anatomical reference if needed).

2. Ask the patient to contract the muscle while you palpate, verifying the location of the muscle.

3. Teach the patient to isolate the muscle by reducing incidental motions and by requesting decreasing muscular effort.

4. Teach the patient minimal contraction effort. (Do not insert the needle until you are successful.) If the patient cannot achieve minimal isolated contraction of this muscle, start somewhere else.

D. Exam Method

1. Ask the patient to contract the muscle, re-identify the muscle by palpation, and locate the point you plan to insert the electrode. Straddle the point with two fingers of your hand.

2. Tell the patient to relax—wait until he or she does—then press down with the fingers and spread the skin (tighten). Touch the skin with the needle (hold at a 45-degree angle). Turn on the patient input of the preamplifier. From this point on, the sound is important and should be on. Press through the skin with a quick, short thrust. Penetrate the skin quickly.

3. Use the sound as a guide to where you are and what the patient's status is (eg, relaxed and quiet or tense and noisy).

4. Achieve silence (patient relaxed, no contractions). As you advance the needle, listen for normal insertion activity. Use short, quick thrusts to advance the needle.

5. Ask the patient to contract easily. Listen to and look at the units. If they are "close" units, verify your location by asking the patient to make isolated easy contractions of the muscle you are seeking and its nearby neighbors. Do not allow strong contractions when you are attempting to isolate a muscle.

6. When you have proven your location, begin collecting the following data. Do it in your head while you are performing the test of that muscle. Write it down after you have removed the needle.

    a. Insertion activity

    b. Spontaneous activity (patient at rest)

    c. Motor unit configuration (all factors of importance)

    d. Motor unit recruitment (interference pattern)

7. Remove the needle.

8. Move on to the next muscle and repeat the above steps.

9. Follow laboratory procedures for disposal of needle electrodes at the completion of the session.

CASE HISTORY 5

| Table 3-14 | EMG Results of Case 5 | | | | | | | |

Median Nerve

Anatomic Site	Latency (ms)		Distance (cm)		Amplitude (mV)		NCV (m/sec)	
	L	R	L	R	L	R	L	R
Wrist	3.8		8.0		6			
Elbow	8.1		22.0		6		57	
Upper Arm	10.4		12.5		6		54	
Sensory II	3.0		14.0		30μV			

HISTORY

The patient is a 62-year-old woman who works in retail sales and leads an active life of walking daily and gardening. She was admitted to the hospital with the complaint of recent onset of weakness, especially in the limb girdles, more pronounced in the pelvic girdle region. She also complains of a general feeling of malaise and was developing a skin rash.

PHYSICAL EXAMINATION

Manual muscle testing reveals significant weakness in the limb girdles with muscle test grades of 2+/5 in the hip flexors, abductors, and extensors, and 3-/5 in the hip rotators. Grades of 2+/5 are also obtained in the shoulder flexors, abductors, internal and external rotators, and triceps. Distal extremity strength is normal. The patient has a positive Trendelenburg sign bilaterally and complains of rapid fatigue on limb girdle activity. No sensory loss is noted and deep tendon reflexes are equal and active at all sites. Functionally, the patient has great difficulty with ambulation unless assisted and using a walker. The patient also cannot perform tasks requiring her to reach over her head. The patient's rash has developed a "butterfly" distribution over the face and is much more noticeable in the trunk and limb girdle areas, and is diminished or absent over the distal aspects of the limbs (Tables 3-14, 3-15, and 3-16).

Table 3-15

EMG Results of Case 5

Ulnar Nerve

	Latency (msec)		Distance (cm)		Amplitude (mV)		NCV (m/sec)	
Anatomic Site	L	R	L	R	L	R	L	R
Wrist	3.0		8.0		10			
Elbow	6.7		21.5		105		8	
Upper Arm	9.0		16.0		10		70	
Sensory II	2.6		14.0		25 µV			

Table 3-16

EMG Results

Muscles Tested	Spontaneous Activity	Potentials Seen on Volition	Recruitment and Interference Pattern
Upper Extremity			
Deltoid (anterior and middle portion)	Fibrillation and sharp waves persistent	AMU-short duration low amplitude, and SLAP potential	Full interference Pattern with moderate effort
Lateral triceps	Fibrillations	Same as above	Same as above
Sternocleidomastoid	0	Same as above	Same as above
Extensor carpi radialis	0	NMU, few AMU	Normal
First dorsal interosseous		NMU, occasional polyphasic potential	Normal
Lower Extremity			
Iliopsoas	Fibrillations and sharp waves, repetitive discharge	AMU, SLAP	Full interference pattern with moderate effort
Gluteus medius	0	AMU, SLAP	Same as above
Gluteus maximus	0	AMU SLAP	Same as above
Tibialis anterior	0	AMU and NMU equal number	Normal
Extensor digitorum brevis	0	NMU	Normal

SLAP = short-duration low-amplitude polyphasic potential
NMU = normal motor unit
AMU = abnormal motor unit

SUMMARY

The electrophysiologic testing in this patient shows that the peripheral nerves on conduction velocity testing were unaffected, but the EMG reveals marked abnormalities that were compatible with a myopathic disorder. These myopathic changes were the most severe in the proximal limb muscles making up the limb girdles.

The clinical electrophysiologic testing combined with the clinical and laboratory examination helped the referring physician arrive at the diagnosis of dermatomyositis.

CASE HISTORY 6

Referring Diagnoses: R/O nerve root compression, L4 through S1, left. lower extremity

Referred by: *Date:*

Problem: Low back and left buttock pain

HISTORY

The patient is a 44-year-old male who works as a postal supervisor. He has an 8-year history of periodic episodes of low back pain with radiation of pain into the buttock and posterior and lateral thigh. The patient states that the current episode began 4 weeks ago and that pain had become severe in the low back, buttock, and posterolateral thigh. He ambulates with a cane and maintains a semiflexed posture.

PHYSICAL EXAMINATION

The patient ambulates with a cane, posture is forward flexed. He moves from standing to sitting and returns to standing very cautiously.

Palpation

The patient has marked tenderness over L4 and L5 spinous processes. Marked muscle spasm was noted bilaterally in the lumbar area, more prominent on the left.

Range of Motion

Forward flexion is severely limited and painful, lateral flexion to the right is normal. Lateral flexion to the left could not be done due to pain. Extension is also painful and severely limited.

Neurological

Ankle jerk (AJ) reflex on the left is decreased compared to right, knee jerk (KJ) reflexes are present and equal bilaterally. The patient has decreased response to pin prick over the dorsum of the foot and lateral border of the foot.

Special Tests

Straight leg raise (SLR) on the left was positive at 40 degrees for radiation to posterior knee. On the right, negative SLR caused low back pain at 70 degrees. The patient has a markedly positive bowstring test on the left. Patrick test causes mild hip pain and increased low back pain.

Table 3-17

EMG Exam

Muscles Tested	Spontaneous Activity	Activity on Volition	Recruitment and Interference Pattern
Vastus lateralis L2, L3	0	NMU	Normal
Vastus medialis L3, L4	0	NMU	Normal
Adductor magnus L2-L4	0	NMU	Normal
Tibialis anterior L4, L5	0	NMU, large MU up to 10 mV, 30% polyphasic potentials	Decreased by 50%
Peroneus longus L5, S1	0	NMU, large MU 6 mV, few polyphasic potentials	Decreased by 50%
Extensor digitorum longus L5, S1	0	NMU, large MU 6 mV, few polyphasic potentials	Decreased by 50%
Extensor digitorum brevis	0	NMU, large MU 20 mV, abnormal MU also mixed with polyphasic potentials	Decreased by 40%
Medial and lateral gastrocnemius S1, S2	0	NMU	Normal
Soleus S2, S2	0	NMU, 30% polyphasic potentials	Marked decrease, single MU pattern

NMU= normal motor unit

NERVE CONDUCTION VELOCITY EXAMINATION

Normal femoral, tibial, and peroneal nerves on MNCV testing, H reflex testing bilaterally revealed a prolonged H latency on the left by 2.4 ms compared to the right (see Chapter 4 for explanation of H reflex testing) (Table 3-17).

ASSESSMENT

EMG abnormalities are primarily of a chronic nature as shown by the distribution of large motor units and decreased interference patterns in the muscles that are supplied by L5 nerve root. In addition, the patient shows abnormal numbers of polyphasic potentials in the same L5 nerve root distribution that may be indicative of more recent and acute changes. The H reflex being delayed as well as the findings in the soleus muscle indicate involvement of the S1 nerve root as well.

COMMENTARY

EMG and NCV testing in nerve root pathology cannot precisely localize the site of nerve root compression. Imaging studies are needed for that purpose. However, only the EMG study can tell you the physiological status of the involved nerve root. The combination of EMG/NCV studies with imaging studies is superior to either, when done separately, in evaluating a patient's nerve root pathology.

Review Questions

1. Describe the basic physiologic principles on which the electromyographic examination is based.

2. Describe (a) the characteristics of a normal motor unit, and (b) the expected findings in normal EMG examination.

3. Discuss the general procedure of planning and conducting an EMG examination.

4. What are the characteristics of (a) a fibrillation potential, and (b) a positive sharp wave? When are they likely to be found?

5. How can you distinguish between fibrillation potentials and motor end-plate potentials?

6. Describe the characteristics of a polyphasic potential. What is the significance of these potentials?

7. If a motor unit potential is larger than normal, what does this indicate?

8. Describe other changes in a motor unit's characteristics that may indicate the motor unit is abnormal.

9. Do myotonic potentials indicate that a patient has a myotonic disease? Explain your answer.

10. What EMG abnormalities are found in myopathic disorders? Discuss the rationale for these findings.

11. Describe methods of confirming your needle location in muscle (ie, identify the muscle) when doing an EMG exam.

chapter 4

Second Waveforms

OBJECTIVES

At the end of this unit of study the reader will be able to:

✧ Describe the characteristics of the F wave and H wave and define the difference between the two responses.

✧ Perform an F wave latency examination of the ulnar and median nerves.

✧ Perform an F wave examination that results in an axillary F central latency (AFCL).

✧ Describe the use of the F wave and AFCL, and use the nomograms for F waves to define upper extremity clinical problems.

✧ Perform an H wave test on the tibial nerve for the purpose of doing an S1 nerve root examination.

✧ Describe the usefulness of this examination and how to use the nomograms for determining the results of an examination.

Table 4-1 COMPARISON OF F WAVE AND H RESPONSE

	F Wave	H Response
Response	Not a reflex, antidromic motor discharge	Monosynaptic
Pathway	Alpha motor fibers	IA sensory, alpha motor
Stimulus	Supramaximal (absent with submaximal stimulus)	Subthreshold (absent with supramaximal stimulus)
Persistence	Variable	Constant with low rates of stimulation
Latency	Variable	Constant, shorter than F wave
Amplitude	Usually small, 5% of M maximum	50 to 100% of maximum M wave, much larger than F wave
Able to test (muscles to record from)	Almost every distal muscle	Gastrocsoleus (tibial nerve in adult), hands-feet intrinsics in children

F Wave—Basic Information

The F wave was first described by Magladery and McDougal in 1950. The F wave can be recorded from the intrinsic muscles of the hands and feet most easily, but F waves can also be recorded from any skeletal muscle. Special stimulation techniques are required to record F waves from proximal muscles in the extremities because the usual techniques for performing conduction studies would tend to obscure the F wave in the MAP.

In their original investigation, Magladery and McDougal called the waveform the F wave. Why this name was given for this second, or later, waveform is not clear, but the presumed answer is that they originally recorded it from the intrinsic muscles of the foot.

Many of the initial investigations of the waveform were directed at determining if the response was an antidromic motor response or whether there was a reflex component. The evidence over several studies has demonstrated the motor antidromic impulse as the source of the wave.

Initial enthusiasm about the clinical use of the F wave was mixed. After a limited number of studies conducted in clinical situations, the usefulness of the F wave has been established.

The F wave is not a reflex and no synapse with another axon or nerve cell is involved. The explanation for the F wave is that with supramaximal stimulation the antidromic wave that is carried back to the anterior horn cells will be "turned around" by a small number of these cells at the axon hillock and then descend the axon as an orthodromic wave and cause a late arriving small second wave (Table 4-1, Figures 4-1 and 4-2).

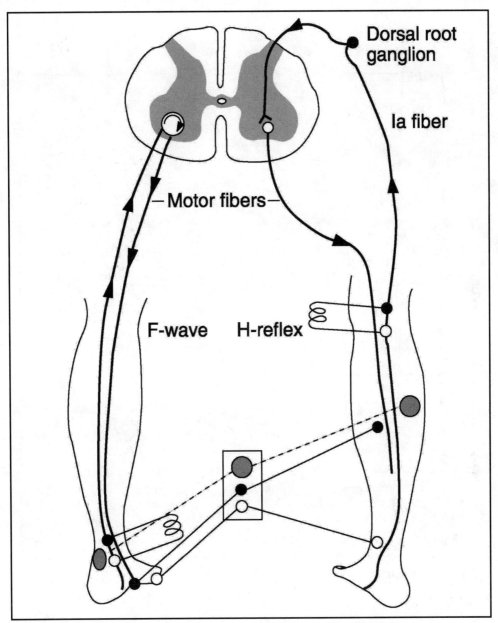

Figure 4-1. Illustration showing the origin of F waves and the H reflex.

F wave studies supplement the routine NCV and EMG studies and have been found to be most useful in clinical conditions where the most proximal portion of the axon is involved. These conditions are:

1. Guillain-Barré syndrome
2. Thoracic outlet syndrome

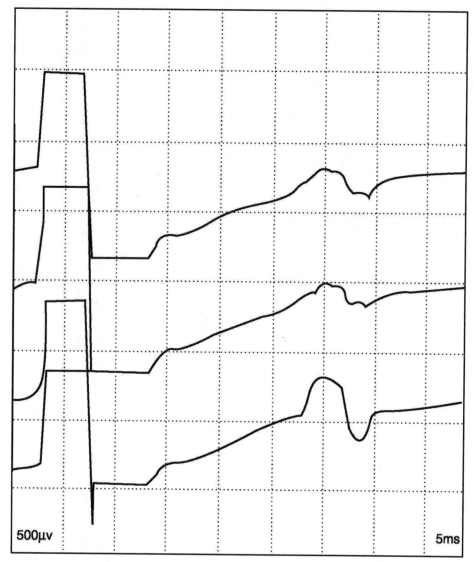

Figure 4-2. Example of an F wave recording.

3. Brachial and lumbosacral plexus lesions (injuries)
4. Sciatic nerve lesions (injuries) at the intragluteal level
5. Radiculopathies if multiple (eg, two or more) nerve roots are involved

There are three ways information can be derived from F wave studies. The first is the F latency, which is the total time from stimulus to F wave initial defection and includes, within it, the M wave latency. A second method is to compute an F conduction time, which is the F latency (ms) – M latency (ms) ÷ 2. This method is not frequently used but contributes data for computing an F velocity. The third way, the

F velocity (m/sec), is found by measuring from the site of stimulation to the C7 spinous process in millimeters and dividing this by the F conduction time. This technique is useful in the upper extremities only.

F latencies are the most frequently used information for F wave studies (see nomograms as examples). See Table 4-1 for comparison of the F wave and H wave.

A method to study the more proximal portion of the F wave has been proposed and is based on defining an axillary F central pathway (Figure 4-3). The conduction time on this pathway is called the axillary F central latency (AFCL). This method has been applied to proximal lesions such as thoracic outlet syndrome, cervical spine radiculopathies (two or more nerve roots), and brachial plexus lesions. Laboratory Exercise 10 will lead the student through the techniques and use of a formula for completing the AFCL.

Bibliography

Braddom RL, Johnson E. Standardization of H reflex and diagnostic use in S radiculopathy. *Arch Phys Med Rehabil*. 1975; 55-166.

Dimitru D. Special nerve conduction techniques. In: Dimitru D, ed. *Electrodiagnostic Medicine*. Philadelphia, Pa: Hanley and Belfus; 1995:177-209.

Kimura J. The F wave, and H, T, Masseter and other reflexes. In: Kimura J, ed. *Electrodiagnosis in Diseases of Muscle and Nerve*. 2nd ed. Philadelphia, Pa: FA Davis; 1989:332-352,356-374.

Lachman T, Shabani BT, Young RR: Late responses as aids to diagnosis in peripheral neuropathy. *Journal of Neurology, Neurosurgery and Psychiatry*. 1980; 43:156-162.

Magladery JW, McDougal DB: Electrophysiologic studies of nerve and reflex activities in normal man & identification of certain reflexes in the electromyogram and conduction velocity of peripheral nerve fibers. *Bull Johns Hopkins Hosp*. 1950; 86:265-290.

Mysieu JW. Late responses: The H, F, and A waves. In: Johnson EW, Pease WS, eds. *Practical Electromyography*. 3rd ed. Baltimore, Md: Williams and Wilkins; 1997.

Weber RJ, Piero DL. F wave evaluation of thoracic outlet syndrome: a multiple regression derived F wave latency predicting technique. *Arch Phys Med Rehabil*. 1997;59:464-469.

Wu Y, Kunz JKM, Putnam ED, Stratigos JS. Axillary F central latency: simple electrodiagnostic techniques for proximal neuropathy. *Arch Phys Med Rehabil*. 1983:64:117-120.

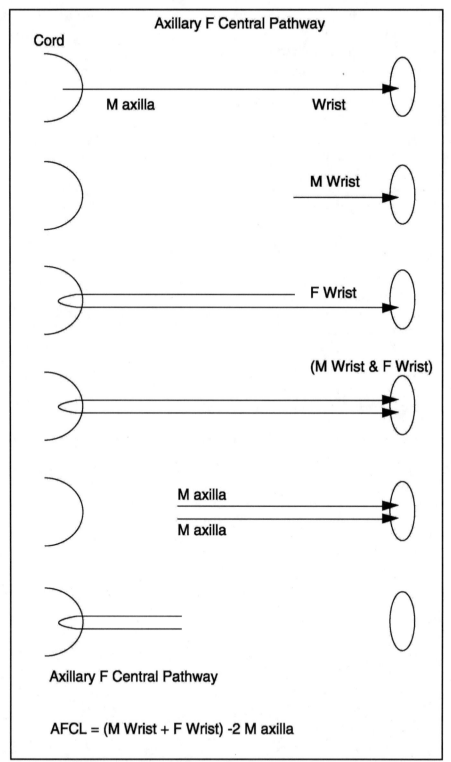

Figure 4-3. Axillary F central pathway.

LABORATORY EXERCISE 10
F Wave

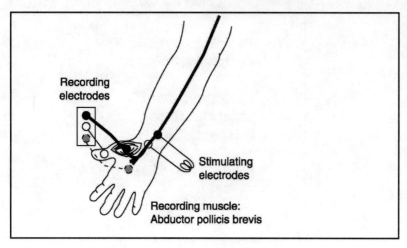

Recording electrodes

Stimulating electrodes

Recording muscle: Abductor pollicis brevis

Figure 4-4. Recording the F wave from the median nerve.

OBJECTIVE

At the conclusion of this laboratory exercise the reader will be able to perform an F wave latency and an AFCL study of the ulnar and median nerves.

A. Set up the EMG machine for F wave study.

   1. Sensitivity: 200 or 500 µV/div

   2. Sweep: 5 ms/div

   3. Stimulus

      a. Rate: 1/sec

      b. Duration: 0.1 ms

   4. Filters—MNCV—Frequency response 2 Hz to 10 kHz (same as MNCV studies)

B. Subject positioning

   1. For F latency of ulnar and/or median nerve: supine with arm comfortably at the side in 30-degree abduction.

   2. For AFCL: supine with arm abducted to 90 degrees and fully supported.

C. Electrode placement

   1. Recording, reference, and ground electrode placements for all major motor nerves are exactly as they were described earlier for conducting MNCV studies.

   2. Stimulating electrode placemement

      a. Distal sites of stimulation for MNCV studies are the most common sites for stimulation. Electrode position is reversed (eg, negative pole proximal instead of distal) (Figure 4-4).

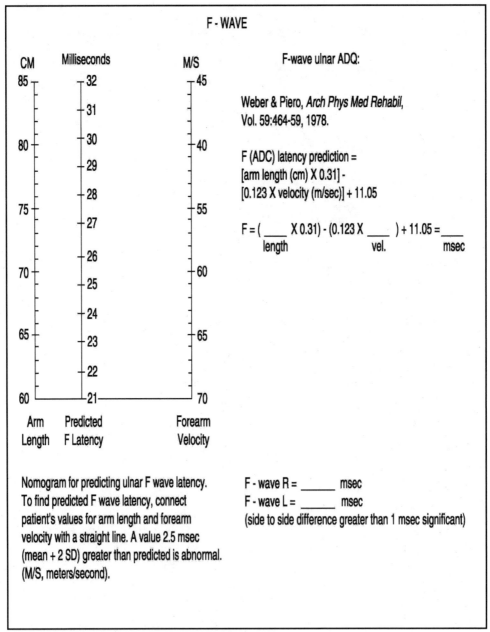

Figure 4-5. Nomogram for F wave study of the ulnar nerve.

b. If computing an F velocity for a segment, for example, stimulation of the ulnar and median nerve sites at the elbow and upper arm can be done.

D. F wave latency technique for the ulnar and median nerves (Figures 4-5 and 4-6)

1. Stimulate at the wrist site so that 10 F waves are seen. Count the number of stimuli required to see 10 F waves.

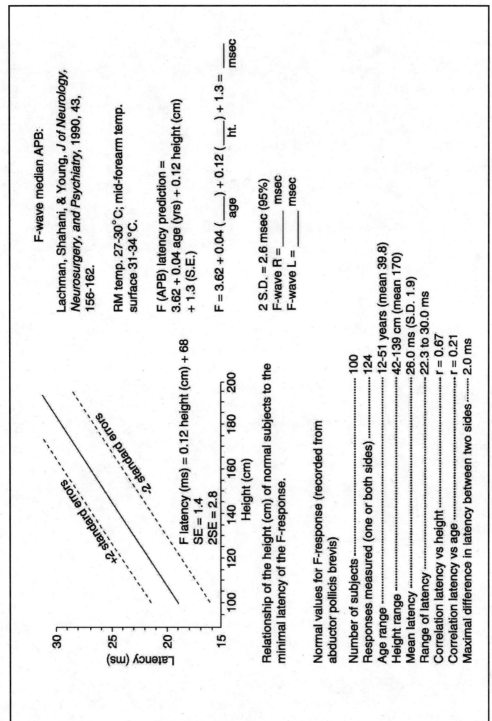

F-wave median APB:

Lachman, Shahani, & Young, *J of Neurology, Neurosurgery, and Psychiatry,* 1990, 43, 156-162.

RM temp. 27-30°C; mid-forearm temp. surface 31-34°C.

F (APB) latency prediction = 3.62 + 0.04 age (yrs) + 0.12 height (cm) + 1.3 (S.E.)

$$F = 3.62 + 0.04 \, (\underline{\quad}) + 0.12 \, (\underline{\quad}) + 1.3 = \underline{\quad} \text{msec}$$
$$\qquad\qquad\qquad\quad \text{age} \qquad\quad \text{ht.}$$

2 S.D. = 2.6 msec (95%)
F-wave R = _____ msec
F-wave L = _____ msec

F latency (ms) = 0.12 height (cm) + 68
SE = 1.4
2SE = 2.8

Height (cm)

Latency (ms)

Relationship of the height (cm) of normal subjects to the minimal latency of the F-response.

Normal values for F-response (recorded from abductor pollicis brevis)

Number of subjects	100
Responses measured (one or both sides)	124
Age range	12-51 years (mean 39.8)
Height range	42-139 cm (mean 170)
Mean latency	26.0 ms (S.D. 1.9)
Range of latency	22.3 to 30.0 ms
Correlation latency vs height	r = 0.67
Correlation latency vs age	r = 0.21
Maximal difference in latency between two sides	2.0 ms

Figure 4-6. Nomogram for F wave study of the median nerve.

2. Use the storage capability of the EMG machine so that the shortest latency seen of the 10 F waves is recorded.

3. Measure arm length from the C7 spinous process to the tip of the ulnar styloid process (arm abducted 30 degrees and palm facing forward [forearm supinated] for ulnar nerve. For the median nerve, follow the same procedure except the forearm should be pronated and the measurement is to the radial styloid process).

E. F wave technique for AFCL of the ulnar and median nerves

1. Stimulate at the wrist and record M latency.

2. Stimulate at the wrist and record F latency as described above.

3. Measure from the sternal notch to the axilla a distance of 25 cm and stimulate here to record an M latency (axilla site).

4. Calculate the AFCL from the formula AFCL = (Mw + Fw)–2 x max. (see Figure 4-3).

F. Expected results

1. AFCL = 11.2 + SD 0.8 ms. A difference of greater than 2.1 ms (approximately 2.5 SD) for nerve-to-nerve in the same extremity or side-to-side comparisons is considered abnormal.

2. For F latency use the nomogram and compare expected to obtained F latency based on nomogram (see Figures 4-5 and 4-6).

H Wave—Basic Information

The H wave (reflex, response) was originally described by Hoffman in 1918 and re-examined by Magladery who named it the H reflex in 1950. The terms H wave and H reflex are used interchangeably. The H wave is considered to represent a monosynaptic reflex response of the Ia afferent fibers of the muscle spindle, which synapse with alpha motor neurons that provide the efferent limb of the reflex. There remains a controversy about where and how easily the H wave can be elicited in adult subjects. The H wave is most easily and consistently elicited from the S1 nerve roots and the tibial nerve in adults. The H wave can be elicited easily from other nerves in infants.

Interest in the H wave can also be attributed to the study in 1950 of Magladery and McDougal, who in effect "rediscovered" the H reflex and rekindled interest in it.

The history of studies done on this wave is similar in some ways to the F wave in that establishing a reliable clinical usefulness was a major area of investigation. Also, the H wave has become of interest to neurophysiologists in research areas because it is a way to demonstrate changes or effects of various activities on a monosynaptic reflex.

The most common clinical use of the H wave is in examination of the S1 nerve root in patients with suspected nerve root irritation or compression accompanying low back pain and radiating pain in one or both lower extremities. Table 4-1 shows the differences between the F wave and H wave.

General factors to consider in the technique to elicit the H wave:

✧ Use a submaximal stimulus to evoke a response. The M wave should be very small or absent in comparison to the H wave.

✧ Supramaximal stimulus obliterates the H wave.

✧ The H wave can be facilitated by mild stretch or mild contraction of the muscle from which a response is being recorded.

✧ Stimulation rates of faster than 1/sec inhibit the response—clinical stimulation at the rate of 1 every 2 sec is recommended.

LABORATORY EXERCISE 11
Clinical EMG Techniques

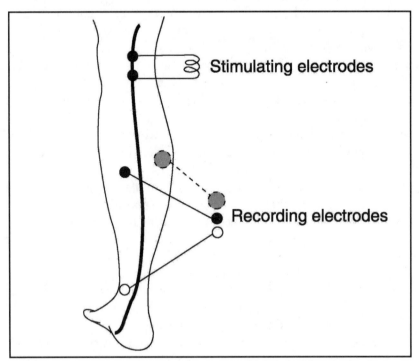

Figure 4-7. Electrode placement for recording the H reflex in the S1 nerve root.

OBJECTIVE

At the conclusion of this laboratory exercise the reader will be able to perform an examination for eliciting the H wave from the gastrocnemius-soleus muscle group (S1 nerve root).

A. Set up the EMG machine for H reflex study

  1. Sensitivity: 500 mV/div to 2 mV/div (depends on response)

  2. Sweep: 5 ms/div

  3. Stimulus

   a. Rate: 1 every 2 sec (.05/sec)

   b. Duration: 0.1 ms

   c. Intensity: submaximal (critical factor)

  4. Filters—same as for MNCV—2 Hz to 10 kHz

B. Subject positioning

   1. Prone position—be sure that the leg is supported but that plantarflexion at the ankle is not inhibited.

C. Electrode placement (Figure 4-7)

   1. Recording electrode (negative)—placement is determined by measuring from the mid-popliteal space to the proximal point on the medial malleolus just as it rises to a prominence. Divide this distance in half and place the electrode at the junction of the upper and lower half of measurement.

   2. Reference electrode (positive)—placed over the Achilles' tendon.

   3. Ground electrode—placed over the mid-calf lateral to the recording electrode and approximately midway between recording and reference electrodes.

D. H wave technique—gastrocnemius-soleus muscle group (S1 nerve root)

   1. Stimulate at the popliteal space—essentially the same as stimulating the tibial nerve to perform MNCV testing. Advance intensity of stimulus slowly and carefully—observe for an H wave with minimal to no MAP. Stimulus must be submaximal.

   2. Measure latency to H wave (initial deflection of waveform).

   3. Calculate predicted H wave latency from the following formula: H latency (ms) = 9.14 + 0.46___(leg length) (cm) + 0.1___(age in years).

   4. Compare the obtained H wave latency to the H wave latency predicted from the formula, or use the nomogram (Figures 4-8 and 4-9).

E. Interpretation of results of the H wave study of the S1 nerve root

   1. Standard deviation (SD) of side-to-side comparison is 0.4 ms, 3 SD = 1.2, therefore if the side-to-side difference is greater than 1 ms it strongly indicates an S1 nerve root involvement.

   2. Steps for evaluation of the H wave of the S1 nerve root:

     a. If obtained H latency is greater than predicted H latency, do contralateral side and then compare as above

     b. If both obtained H latencies are greater than predicted H latency, do MNCV studies of the tibial nerve bilaterally to help evaluate whether the patient has peripheral neuropathy

     c. Prolonged H wave latency is more valuable than an absent H wave latency in interpretation of S1 nerve root pathology

The nomogram developed by Braddom and Johnson relates H latency to leg length and age using the formula on the previous page (Figure 4-8).

The nomogram by Lachman, Shahani, and Young (1980) relates height to measured latency using the formula below (Figure 4-9):

H latency (ms)=2.74 + 0.05–age in years + 0.14 (height in cm) + 1.4 (1 SE*)

*1 standard error

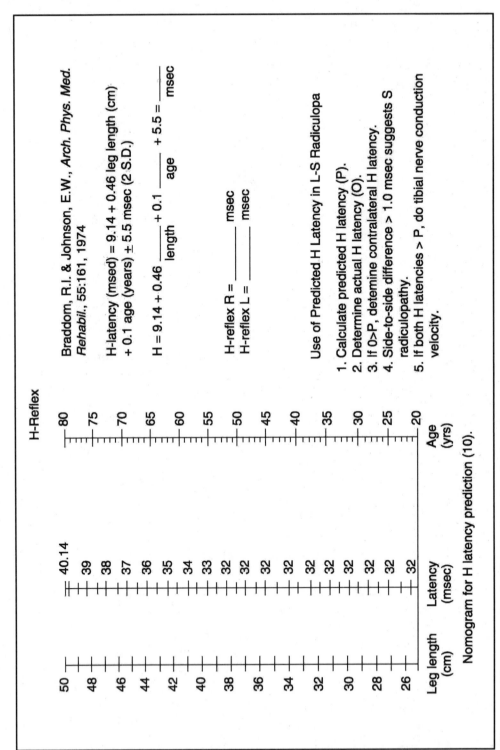

Figure 4-8. Nomogram for the H reflex based on leg length.

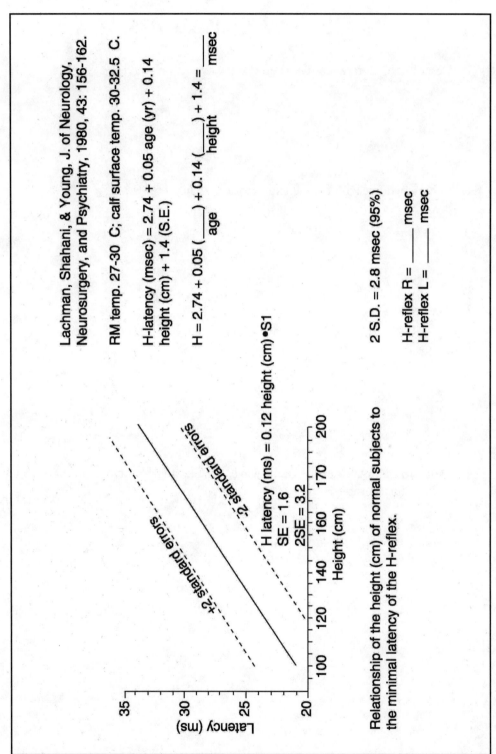

Lachman, Shahani, & Young, J. of Neurology, Neurosurgery, and Psychiatry, 1980, 43: 156-162.

RM temp. 27-30 C; calf surface temp. 30-32.5 C.

H-latency (msec) = 2.74 + 0.05 age (yr) + 0.14 height (cm) + 1.4 (S.E.)

$$H = 2.74 + 0.05 \left(\frac{}{age} \right) + 0.14 \left(\frac{}{height} \right) + 1.4 = \underline{\hspace{1cm}} msec$$

H latency (ms) = 0.12 height (cm)•S1
SE = 1.6
2SE = 3.2

+2 standard errors
-2 standard errors

Height (cm)

Latency (ms)

Relationship of the height (cm) of normal subjects to the minimal latency of the H-reflex.

2 S.D. = 2.8 msec (95%)

H-reflex R = _____ msec
H-reflex L = _____ msec

Figure 4-9. Nomogram for the H reflex based on height.

Review Questions

1. Describe the differences between the F wave and H wave.

2. Outline when each of these examinations would be used.

3. Define:
   a. AFCL
   b. F latency

4. Describe the usefulness of the F wave, AFCL, and H wave examinations as well as the limitations.

5. Define how the H wave examination of the tibial nerve is related to the S1 nerve root.

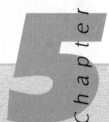

Electromyographic Decision Guide

OBJECTIVES

By using this electromyographic decision guide the reader will be able to:

❖ Describe the importance of and plan the clinical examination of the patient prior to testing.

❖ Plan the basic electrophysiologic examinations for the most commonly referred orthopedic problems, including nerve root compression syndromes and peripheral nerve entrapment syndromes.

❖ Plan the basic electrophysiologic examination for many of the most common neurologic problems, including neuropathies, spinal cord and mixed upper and lower motor nerve diseases, and other neurologic problems.

❖ Plan the basic electrophysiologic examinations for patients with suspected myopathic disorders.

Introduction

The purpose of preparing a decision guide in electromyography (clinical electro-physiologic testing) is to assist the beginning electromyographer by providing a guide to the basic electrophysiologic examination needed for a variety of common problems. Over the years, working with practitioners who are learning electromyography, it seemed obvious that assistance of this type might be beneficial. It may not be possible to provide a complete decision guide but if certain principles concerning the electrophysiologic examination are kept in mind, this guide will aid in performing these tests.

Clinical information derived from the patient's history and clinical examination are of the utmost importance in understanding and defining the amount of electromyographic and nerve conduction velocity testing that needs to be done.

Common sense is a partial guide. If after completing the electrophysiologic testing the patient's clinical findings and the test results do not fit well together, then it is time to re-evaluate the situation and make a decision about what else should be done.

Clinicians cannot expect to do adequate electrophysiologic testing without keeping abreast of the literature and without keeping their understanding of the conditions that they are examining up to date.

In devising a decision guide, I have made the following arbitrary divisions for the guide:

1. *Orthopedic problems*: This primarily includes overuse and entrapment syndromes, plexus injuries and nerve root problems.

2. *Neurologic problems*: Included are neuropathies of all types except overuse and entrapment syndromes (eg, toxic, nutritional, and hereditary). Also included are spinal cord, mixed upper and lower motor neuron lesions, and other neurological conditions such as myotonias and heredofamilial degenerative diseases of the central nervous system.

3. *Myopathies*: Included in this last category are myopathic syndromes, including primary muscle diseases and myasthenic syndromes.

Orthopedic Problems

1. Lumbar spine

   A. Suspected herniated disc—lumbar spine with nerve root pathology.

      a. Routine exam—a minimum of eight muscles in one lower extremity.

         Ex: L2-S2 nerve root distribution (vastus lateralis, vastus medialis, tibialis anterior, extensor digitorum longus, fibularis [peroneus] longus, extensor digitorum brevis, medial and lateral heads of the gastrocnemius)

      b. H reflex wave (for suspected S1 nerve root lesions).

      c. If all muscles involved are fibular (peroneal) nerve distribution (eg, L5 nerve root):

  i. Do other L5 nerve root muscles such as biceps femoris, gluteus maximus, and extensor hallucis longus.

  ii. NCV testing—fibular (peroneal), tibial, and sural nerve—when neuropathy should be ruled out.

B. If sciatic pain is bilateral:

  a. Test most symptomatic leg, as above, first.

  b. Screen opposite extremity, vastus medialis, tibialis anterior, fibularis (peroneus) longus, extensor digitorum brevis, medial gastrocnemius. If full exam is warranted, complete routine.

C. Erector spinae muscles are tested:

  a. Early in the course of the patient's problem

  b. When the extremity pattern does not clearly identify nerve root

  c. If obvious atrophy of erector spinae muscles exists

  d. If the examiner feels this is important to clarify whether the problem is nerve root, plexus, or peripheral nerve.

2. Cervical spine

A. Routine exam. Example: suspected herniated disc or other space-occupying lesion-causing nerve root pathology. Eleven muscles of the upper extremity C5-T2 nerve roots (anterior deltoid, middle deltoid, biceps [both heads], brachioradialis, extensor carpi radialis longus, flexor carpi radialis, extensor carpi ulnaris, extensor pollicis longus, first dorsal interosseous, abductor pollicis brevis, abductor digiti minimi).

B. If the nerve root pattern is not evident but peripheral nerve distribution is, add NCV (motor and sensory) of major nerves: ulnar, radial, median, etc.

C. If there is a question of brachial plexus versus nerve root pathology either by history or distribution of abnormality, do posterior cervical spinal muscles.

D. Add additional muscles (triceps, brachialis, etc) if needed to clarify exam.

E. If symptoms are bilateral, screen extremity with least involvement (middle deltoid, biceps, extensor carpi radialis longus, flexor carpi radialis, abductor pollicis brevis, first dorsal interosseous, others if needed).

3. Entrapment syndromes

A. Carpal tunnel syndrome—routine exam

  a. Motor nerve conduction velocity—ulnar and median nerves. Keep distal distances (site of stimulation to recording electrode) approximately equal (suggest 8 to 10 cm).

  b. Sensory nerve conduction—distal segment ulnar and median nerves (for median nerve do both second and third digits).

  c. EMG of abductor pollicis brevis, first dorsal interosseous, abductor digiti minimi, flexor carpi radialis as minimum exam (do median and ulnar nerves supplied muscles of forearm).

    d. Expand exam if results of nerve conduction velocity are unexpected, especially:

        i. "Cross" stimulation for anastomosis between the ulnar and median nerves.

        ii. If problem seems to be more than entrapment, do expanded EMG exam (eg, plexus or "double crush" problem).

B. Deep branch radial nerve entrapment (radial tunnel syndrome)

    a. Routine exam—radial nerve—stimulate at forearm, elbow, upper arm, supraclavicular for radial nerve conduction velocity.

    b. Sensory nerve conduction—radial nerve (abnormal helps rule out deep branch entrapment).

    c. EMG—extensor pollicis longus, extensor indicis proprius and proximal muscles, extensor carpi radialis longus, brachioradialis, lateral head of triceps.

C. Ulnar nerve compression—elbow

    a. Motor nerve conduction velocity—ulnar and median nerves. Segments of the ulnar nerve across elbow—standardize exam by positioning patient with shoulder abducted to 90 degrees and elbow flexed to 90 degrees, and use minimum of 10 cm segment across the elbow and for the segment above this.

    b. Sensory nerve conduction—ulnar and median nerve.

    c. EMG sample of ulnar and median nerves, both forearm and hand.

D. Femoral nerve entrapment—inguinal area

    a. Motor nerve conduction velocity-femoral nerve, include segment across the inguinal area (use criteria of 1.1 ms difference from above the inguinal ligament to the femoral triangle unless the segment is at least 10 cm). Also compute velocities for longest segments (above inguinal ligament to adductor canal, and femoral triangle to adductor canal) and compare velocities.

    b. EMG—quadriceps (femoral nerve distribution) and sample of other lower extremity muscles for comparison.

    c. Other nerves for motor nerve conduction velocity if above does not clearly indicate problem.

    d. Lateral femoral cutaneous nerve—sensory nerve conduction for *meralgia paresthesia*. Sensory complaints in anterior and lateral thigh.

E. Fibular (peroneal) nerve—fibular head entrapment

    a. Motor nerve conduction velocity—fibular (peroneal) nerve—do segment from the popliteal space to below the fibular head as well as longer segment. Do tibial nerve for comparison.

b. EMG—sample fibular (peroneal) nerve (proximal and distal muscles) and tibial nerve (proximal and distal muscles).

c. If you suspect neuropathy, do sensory nerve conduction, sural nerve, and superficial fibular (peroneal) nerve.

F. Tarsal tunnel syndrome

a. Motor nerve conduction velocity—fibular (peroneal) and tibial nerves. Latencies from both medial and lateral plantar nerves. Measure distance from the point of stimulation above the tarsal tunnel to the recording electrodes. Do bilateral testing if necessary.

b. Sensory tibial nerve latencies—medial and lateral plantar nerves.

c. EMG—sample tibial nerve—proximal and distal (abductor hallucis and muscles above the tarsal tunnel innervated by the tibial nerve).

G. Thoracic outlet syndrome

a. Not likely to find segmental slowing in the cervical rib or scalenus anterior syndrome. Proximal site of stimulation is often below the site of compression.

b. If the problem is lower (under the clavicle or caused by the pectoralis minor, etc), may find slowing of the segment crossing from above the clavicle to the axilla or upper arm.

c. Motor nerve conduction velocity—ulnar nerve and median nerve at all sites. Do sensory latencies of the ulnar and median nerves.

d. EMG to demonstrate no changes/mild changes in peripheral nerve distribution.

e. Ulnar nerve most likely to be involved in vascular syndromes especially reduction of sensory amplitude.

f. Do F wave latencies and axillary F central latency study.

G. Ulnar nerve—entrapment at the wrist (tunnel of Guyon)

a. Motor nerve conduction velocity of the ulnar nerve—distal latency to abductor digiti minimi and to first dorsal interosseous. Compare to median nerve. Look for difference of more than 1.5 ms between the two recording sites of the ulnar nerve .

b. Sensory nerve conduction—ulnar and median nerve.

c. EMG—distal—intrinsic muscles of the hand compared to muscles innervated by the median and ulnar nerves above the wrist.

Neurologic Problems

1. Facial nerve—Bell's palsy (diabetic and traumatic lesions also possible)
   A. Routine exam to be done as soon as possible after onset.
      a. Nerve conduction velocity—latencies to triangularis, frontalis, orbicularis oris—3.5 to 5.0 ms range normal.
      b. EMG—sample triangularis, orbicularis oris (upper and lower lip) orbicularis oculi, frontalis.
      c. Electrical excitability test—repeat exam frequently during first 3 to 10 days. Do EMG of postauricular muscles if patient can "wiggle" ears.

2. Neuropathy (diabetic, alcoholic, etc)
   A. Suspect patients with loss of ankle jerk bilaterally for lower extremity neuropathy.
   B. Start testing in lower extremity, tibial and peroneal nerve first. Move on to femoral, then ulnar, median, and radial nerves of the upper extremity.
   C. Do sensory test of the sural nerve and superficial peroneal nerve of the lower extremity. Ulnar, median, and possibly radial sensory nerves of the upper extremity (perform others as needed).
   D. Do EMG in suspected neuropathy even if nerve conduction velocity is normal. Sample proximal and distal sites.
   E. Test three extremities as the minimum examination in suspected peripheral neuropathies.
   F. Major causes of neuropathies with examples—a good history and clinical exam are essential:
      a. Toxic—lead, alcohol, drugs
      b. Infectious—Guillain-Barré syndrome
      c. Metabolic—diabetes
      d. Nutritional—severe deficiency disease
      e. Malignancies
      f. Hereditary—Charcot-Marie-Tooth disease
   G. Differentiate on basis of pathology
      a. Axonal dying back neuropathies—alcohol, toxic, and metabolic; increased distal latencies
      b. Demyelinating—Guillain-Barré, diabetes
      c. Vascular—polyarteritis nodosa, localized effects
      d. Chronic—hereditary, severe slowing of NCV, Charcot-Marie-Tooth disease

3. Spinal cord and mixed upper and lower motor neuron lesions

A. In conditions such as amyotrophic lateral sclerosis (ALS) one of the primary features may be fasciculation potentials. These must be found widespread and as a general rule should be found in three out of four extremities examined.

B. In attempting to differentiate ALS from progressive spinal muscular atrophy (PSMA), the amount of lower motor neuron involvement is important. ALS can be differentiated from PSMA best on clinical grounds.

C. Clinically, neither one of these conditions has sensory involvement.

D. Motor nerve conduction velocities remain normal but with decreased amplitudes and normal sensory conduction.

E. In both PSMA and ALS, most abnormal findings are found distally in the extremities and progress proximally.

F. If you were trying to differentiate either of these conditions from a patient with cervical syringomyelia, clinically, you should have profound and severe sensory loss. In syringomyelia, the motor changes are most severe in the intrinsic muscles of the hand and in the muscles of the forearm with less or no involvement of the upper arm and shoulder girdle.

G. Spinal cord compressions are essentially the same as nerve root problems in that you are trying to find a nerve root level. Spinal cord compressions in which there is nerve root involvement may help lead to a localization of the level or portion of the spinal cord that is involved, such as in spinal canal tumors.

H. Studies of evoked potentials in ALS have found the following phenomenon: In normal individuals, as you gradually increase the intensity of the stimulus, the amplitude of the evoked muscle action potential will gradually increase with the intensity of the stimulus. The amplitude of the evoked muscle action potential will gradually increase until finally a maximal stimulus is obtained and no further increase in amplitude occurs. If the increases in intensity are small, the increases in amplitude are small. In ALS, as the stimulus intensity is gradually increased, it does not cause any change in the muscle action potential until a seemingly critical level is reached. Then smaller increases in intensity cause exceptionally large increases in the amplitude of the response. Attempts to evoke an intermediate amplitude cannot be obtained. This phenomena is most likely to be found in muscles that are clinically weak. In some instances it has been described that the muscle behaved in an "all or none" fashion with no significant action potential until a great deal of intensity is used and then a normally large action potential can be obtained.

I. In myotonias, the most characteristic abnormalities are the myotonic potentials. There are some myotonias of a rare, congenital nature in which myotonic potentials are not obtained easily, or at all, but myopathic potentials may be obtained, especially in the limb girdle and temporal and masseter muscles. (the older the patient, the fewer myotonic potentials).

J. In early multiple sclerosis it has been reported that abnormalities can be obtained consisting of primarily polyphasic potentials in a scattered non-nerve root type distribution. As a person's MS progresses and muscles are no longer under voluntary control, you may still obtain polyphasic potentials if you can stimulate the muscle mechanically or otherwise to cause contraction.

K. In Friedreich's ataxia, marked loss of sensory nerve action potential amplitude is found. Motor conduction characteristics may be near normal in the lower extremities. Reduced recruitment of motor units and polyphasic potentials may be obtained in the distribution of muscle weakness prior to loss of muscle control when performing EMG examination.

L. In summary, neurologic conditions:

   a. In most suspected neurological problems it is important to do both NCV and EMG studies (often bilaterally including upper and lower extremities).

   b. In certain neurological conditions, the NCV should remain normal while finding markedly abnormal EMGs.

   c. Evaluation of the patient's clinical condition prior to testing is of the utmost importance in neurological patients.

   d. There are some neuromuscular diseases in which electrophysiologic testing experience is insufficient to provide an explanation of expected findings. In these cases, an understanding of the pathology that occurs should help you predict the type of electrophysiologic changes taking place.

Myopathies

1. In primary muscle disease, it is important that a distribution of the patient's weakness or pseudohypertrophy be noted prior to doing the EMG examination.

2. It is important to understand that finding myopathic potentials does not tell you what type of myopathy the patient has. The distribution of abnormalities is probably a more important clue than the severity of the EMG abnormality.

3. Remember that in myopathies you may find:

   A. Spontaneous activity—fibrillation potentials and sharp waves.

   B. On volition—polyphasic potentials.

   C. Myopathic short-duration potentials of smaller amplitude than normal. The myopathic process may involve the distal axon and the motor endplate.

4. The most common myopathies are those associated with the various forms of muscular dystrophy. Other myopathic conditions are:

A. Sarcoid

B. McCardle's syndrome

C. Thyrotoxic myopathy

D. Some carcinomas

E. Alcoholic myopathy

F. Collagen diseases

5. Myasthenia gravis can be differentiated from the Eaton-Lambert syndrome on the basis of evoked potential studies.

A. These are well summarized in recent texts on EMG/NCV testing. The primary difference is that on repetitive stimuli in myasthenia gravis, there is a diminution in response; while in Eaton-Lambert syndrome, on repetitive stimulation studies there is an initial increase in the amplitude of the response.

B. In both of these conditions, nerve conduction velocities should remain normal.

6. Polymyositis and dermatomyositis are collagen diseases in which there is a mixture of myopathic potentials in the proximal musculature, neuropathic potentials, and occasionally fibrillation potentials spontaneously. The collagen disease process of inflammation of connective tissue can extend to include the distal axon, which then becomes involved in the inflammation and gives you abnormal potentials. The clinical features of the disease are important in making a decision about the patient's problem and the areas for EMG examination.

Summary

This chapter is a decision guide that has been developed for use by the beginning electromyographer. It was developed to assist in the thinking process in planning the electrophysiologic examination. It is not intended to be all-inclusive, as there are many neurological and other conditions that you will not find in this guide that you may be called upon to examine. The attempt of the guide is to keep things as simple as possible, without oversimplifying to the point of leaving out important information in performing EMG and NCV examinations. A simple rule that can be followed is that when doing an EMG examination, you should examine until you find a normal area or until you are satisfied that you understand the patient's problem.

Review Questions

1. Discuss the questions clinicians should ask themselves to decide if they are prepared to examine the patient electrophysiologically.

2. Plan the examination for a patient with a suspected carpal tunnel syndrome.

3. Plan the examination for a patient with a suspected lumbar nerve root problem.

4. Discuss the reasons that might require the examination to be extended to the uninvolved lower extremity.

5. What approach would you use in planning the clinical and electrophysiologic examination of a patient with muscle weakness that was widespread?

6. Discuss the limitations of the electrophysiologic examination in patients with myopathies.

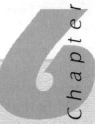

Additional Electrophysiologic Studies

OBJECTIVES

At the end of this unit of study the reader will be able to:

✧ Briefly describe the other nerves in the upper and lower extremities that can be studied using nerve conduction techniques.

✧ Discuss the various technological attempts to improve the objectivity of EMG analysis.

✧ Use the materials suggested in the Suggested Reading to aid in further understanding of the methods described in this section.

✧ Realistically appraise the level of their ability to perform the studies in this manual and determine what more they need to learn to progress as a clinical electrophysiologist.

Future EMG Possibilities

The purpose of this portion of the book is to help users realize that they have examined the basic techniques for doing nerve conduction studies of the most commonly examined nerves and have learned only the basic information about the electromyographic portion of the examination. This chapter will explore some of the other possibilities that exist in the area of clinical electrophysiologic testing and will direct the reader to explore the textbooks cited in the Suggested Reading as sources of information for learning about these additional studies.

Nerve Conduction Velocity Studies (Other Nerves)

UPPER EXTREMITY

There are several other NCV procedures that can be performed. Motor nerve studies can be done on the axillary nerve and on the motor portion of the musculocutaneous nerve. Two techniques have been developed for these two motor nerves. One is to stimulate in the area above the clavicle (supraclavicular) and record latencies to the deltoid in the case of the axillary nerve, and to the biceps for the musculocutaneous nerve. The other method for studying the axillary nerve involves stimulation above the clavicle and at the axilla and computing a velocity on the axillary nerve. The musculocutaneous nerve can be stimulated above the clavicle and then over the musculocutaneous nerve in the upper aspect of the arm at the anterior aspect of the axilla.

Both the long thoracic nerve and the suprascapular nerve can be studied by stimulating the area above the clavicle over the brachial plexus and recording the latencies from the muscles supplied by these nerves; for example, the suprascapular nerve latency to the supraspinatus and infraspinatus and the long thoracic nerve latency to a measured, or preselected, point on the chest from the serratus anterior muscle.

A sensory nerve in the upper extremity that has also been studied is the continuation of the musculocutaneous nerve as the lateral antebrachial cutaneous nerve. This nerve has been studied both orthodromically and antidromically. The medial antebrachial cutaneous nerve has also been studied.

Further information about the nerves of the upper extremity and determining which techniques might be useful can be found in the Suggested Reading after this chapter. Particularly helpful are the texts by Dimitru, Kimura, and Oh.

LOWER EXTREMITY

Sensory nerves that are often examined but are not included in this manual are the saphenous nerve, which can be done both orthodromically and antidromically, and the lateral femoral cutaneous nerve, which is usually done antidromically. However, techniques have been reported for orthodromic stimulation as well. In the lower extremities, the lumbosacral plexus and the sciatic nerve are both deep posteriorly and cannot be studied by conventional stimulation techniques. A variety of techniques have been devised to study the sciatic nerve by inserting needle electrodes for stimulation close to the nerve. Methods have been devised for stimulating individual nerve roots of the lumbosacral plexus using a needle electrode for stimulation inserted close to the nerve root of interest (see Dimitru or Kimura's text for a complete explanation of these techniques).

Two other nerves deserve mentioning, although neither one fits the designation of upper or lower extremity. The first is the spinal accessory nerve (XI cranial nerve), which runs superficially along the posterior border of the sternocleidomastoid muscle. The nerve can be stimulated at this point and a response can be recorded from the upper trapezius. The other nerve is the phrenic nerve. A method of using surface stimulation of the phrenic nerve in the anterior cervical region and recording by surface electrodes from the anterior chest has been found to be useful.

BLINK REFLEX

The blink reflex has been studied electrophysiologically for quite some time. The blink reflex can be recorded using commonly available clinical machines. It has proven to be useful in evaluating patients with involvement of the trigeminal or facial nerve, patients with multiple sclerosis or other brainstem lesions, and patients with a variety of polyneuropathies. A detailed discussion of the study method of the blink reflex is well beyond the intention of this beginners' manual and the reader is referred to other texts in the Suggested Reading.

REPETITIVE STIMULATION STUDIES

Assessment of disorders of the neuromuscular junction and the electrophysiologic evaluation of neuromuscular transmission requires the use of repetitive stimulation and examination of the evoked potentials as a result of this repetitive stimulation. This type of examination has been found useful in Eaton-Lambert syndrome, myasthenia gravis, and other disorders of the neuromuscular junction.

The reader is referred to the Suggested Reading for information concerning these studies. This is a particularly important area in which technique is one of the most critical factors in conducting a study of a patient. An electromyographer attempting to study the neuromuscular junction must have a well-defined protocol in mind and have experience with the use of that protocol.

ELECTROMYOGRAPHY

Several attempts to improve electromyography by various technical methods have been investigated and proposed. Clinical electromyography involves the assessment of motor unit characteristics as displayed on the oscilloscope from which the experienced examiner can then detect the abnormalities with reasonable certainty. Essentially, clinical electromyography, as done in the conventional clinical manner, is the subjective assessment of highly objective data. To remove this subjective assessment portion of the electromyography examination, there has been a number of methods developed in an attempt to improve the certainty and to decrease the subjectivity of the analysis.[1-3]

These quantitative methods have included a variety of approaches. One has been a method to improve the measurement of motor unit characteristics that requires the recording of at least 20 different motor units in each muscle, using multiple needle insertions and then comparing the information gathered to normal values that had been gathered in the same laboratory environment. As is evident, this is a very time-consuming procedure. Other methods of quantifying electromyography have been to examine motor unit territory, methods to estimate motor unit numbers, and frequency analysis. Each of these methods requires a special approach of either altering the electrode system or altering the recording system and expanding the memory of the recording system. Each of these quantitative methods can be demonstrated to show some improvement in the analysis. For example, motor unit territory analysis has demonstrated that the motor unit territory is increased in patients with neurogenic weakness. This increase in territory is presumed to be the result of reinnervation of the denervated muscle fibers by collateral sprouting from surviving axons. In contrast, in patients who suffer primarily from muscle disease, there is a decrease in motor unit territory.

Frequency analysis is a subject that would require a great deal of explanation. Basically, this type of analysis reveals that the shorter the duration of the motor unit potential, the greater the higher frequency components. Subjects with myopathic disorders would have higher frequencies than those with anterior horn cell lesions or peripheral neuropathies.

Two of the concepts that are currently being explored in the area of electromyography are that of single fiber electromyography and so called macroelectromyography (macro EMG). Single fiber electromyography is based on the need to examine not just motor unit activity, but muscle fiber activity within the same motor unit as well. The use of this technique has contributed to the understanding of muscle physiology and pathophysiology. This technique requires the use of a specially designed recording electrode. The interval between the firing of two action potentials within the same motor unit is called the interpotential interval and there is a temporal component referred to as jitter. Measurement of jitter is considered to be a sensitive means of evaluating neuromuscular transmission within a motor unit.

Macro EMG is a technique that has been developed to study the size of motor units and motor unit territories. Conventional electromyography, while providing information about motor unit activity, does not provide complete information about the size of motor units or the territory of motor units. The technique of macro EMG, by using a specially designed electrode and averaging techniques, provides for or allows the contribution of all muscle fibers belonging to a motor unit during voluntary muscle contraction to be recorded. Several factors determine the characteristics of the macro EMG such as the number of fibers, the fiber diameter, the endplate scatter, the pattern of nerve branching, and the motor unit territory.

Both single fiber electromyography and macro EMG are contributing to our understanding of the anatomy and physiology of both healthy and abnormal motor units.[2]

EVOKED POTENTIAL STUDIES

The last area to be discussed is that of evoked potentials. In Appendix B, you will find the definition for *brainstem visual evoked potentials*, and a definition for *brainstem auditory evoked potentials*. These two types of studies have been used extensively in neurology for examining patients for a variety of conditions. The techniques for performing these studies require peripheral equipment in addition to the basic EMG equipment. In visual evoked potential studies, a television monitor with a checker board pattern, which alternates the color of the squares at a regular frequency, is used as the stimulus. Recording is done from the visual cortical area using surface electrodes. The same principle is used in auditory evoked potential studies in which a click generator is used as the stimulus and recordings are made from the cortical areas that have an auditory projection. Both of these types of studies have unique potential characteristics that permit the examiner to make inferences about the visual and/or auditory pathway and the abnormalities encountered in relationship to nervous system pathology.

SOMATOSENSORY POTENTIALS

When doing sensory nerve conduction studies the focus is on the peripheral portion of the nerve. The more proximal segments of sensory nerves are not easily accessible for study. Studies of somatosensory evoked potentials (SEPs) can be used to assess the entire length of the somatosensory pathway. Electrical stimuli are most commonly used and the most common sites of stimulation are the median or ulnar nerve at the wrist, the tibial nerve at the ankle, and the fibular (peroneal) nerve at the knee. In addition, dermatome sites have also been used and standard sites described. The frequency, duration, and number of stimuli depends primarily on the purpose of the study. Recording is done from scalp areas using the international 10 to 20 system that has been used by electroencephalographers for determining where surface electrodes will be placed on the scalp. In addition to surface electrodes placed over the scalp, according to a prearranged plan, responses are also recorded over the spine. An example would be stimulating the median nerve in the upper extremity and recording from the area above the clavicle (supraclavicular) and the C7 and the C2 spinous processes as well as the contralateral hand area of the scalp using a scalp electrode placed at the mid-frontal area. Similar examples can be used for the lower extremity where recording over the L1 and L3 lumbar spines is common when stimulating the fibular (peroneal) nerve at the knee. The higher reference point is also used in the example for the upper extremity. SEPs have been used to examine both peripheral and central nervous systems.

In the clinical context, there has been interest in using SEPs to examine the most proximal parts of peripheral nerves, the plexus and spinal nerve roots. SEPs have been used in the evaluation of brachial plexus injuries, thoracic outlet syndrome, cervical nerve root, and lumbar nerve root lesions. The diagnostic capability of sensory evoked potentials in examining lumbar nerve root lesions has not been found to be as useful as conventional needle electromyography. SEPs have also been used in patients with Guillain-Barré syndrome, which helps to demonstrate pathology in the proximal portion of peripheral nerves when conventional nerve conduction studies remain normal. In addition, somatosensory evoked potentials have been used to evaluate functions of the sensory nervous system. These techniques have been used in patients with suspected multiple sclerosis, and subclinical lesions have been detected. These studies have also been used to evaluate patients with spinal cord injuries and have been useful in both diagnosis and prognosis.[1-3]

Conclusion

This chapter was included simply to inform the beginning clinical electromyographer that there are many possibilities beyond those covered in this introductory text. It was also included to emphasize the importance of using a standard text in learning basic information about the various techniques discussed in this section and also to indicate the complex nature of the types of studies that are developing and being used. This should also help you understand that there is a very large body of literature that needs to be consulted for the latest information on new and developing techniques and their application to various neuromuscular conditions. It is hoped that this section will encourage further study and will help the reader to appreciate the level of challenge that exists in performing clinical electrophysiologic studies.

No review questions are provided for this chapter. The purpose of the chapter was to provide the student with an understanding of the remaining possibilities for further learning and the need for further studies.

References

1. Aminoff M. Quantitative and related techniques and other diagnostic techniques for the evaluation of neuromuscular disorders. In: Aminoff M, ed. *Electromyography in Clinical Practice*. 3rd ed. New York: Churchill-Livingstone; 1998:147-198.
2. Dimitru D. Special nerve conduction techniques, special needle electromyographic techniques, and somatosensory evoked potentials. In: Dimitru D, ed. *Electrodiagnostic Medicine*. Philadelphia, Pa: Hanley and Belfus; 1995:177-209,249-279,281-337.
3. Kimura J. Single fiber and macro electromyography and somatosensory evoked potentials. In: Kimura J, ed. *Electrodiagnosis in Diseases of Muscle and Nerve*. 2nd ed. Philadelphia, Pa: FA Davis; 1986:285-304,375-426.

Suggested Reading

Aminoff MJ. *Electromyography in Clinical Practice.* 3rd ed. NY: Churchill Livingstone; 1998.

Brooke M. *A Clinician's View of Neuromuscular Diseases.* 2nd ed. Baltimore, Md: Williams and Wilkins; 1986.

Currier DP. Electromyography as a clarifying tool. In: Wolf SL, ed. *Electrotherapy.* NY: Churchill Livingstone; 1981.

Dawson DM, Hallett M, Millender LH. *Entrapment Neuropathies.* 3rd ed. Philadelphia, Pa: Lippincott Williams & Wilkins; 1998.

Dimitru D. *Electrodiagnostic Medicine.* Philadelphia, Pa: Hanley and Belfus; 1995.

Dyck L, Dyck T, eds. *Peripheral Neuropathy.* 2nd ed. Philadelphia, Pa: WB Saunders; 1984.

Liveson JA. *Peripheral Neurology: Case Studies in Electrodiagnosis.* 3rd ed. Philadelphia, Pa: Oxford University Press; 2000.

Millender LH, Louis DS, Simmons BP. *Occupational Disorders of the Upper Extremities.* New York: Churchill Livingstone; 1992.

Oh S. *Principles of Clinical Electromyography.* Philadelphia, Pa: Lippincott Williams & Wilkins; 1998.

Omer GE, Spinner M, Van Beek AL. *Management of Peripheral Nerve Problems.* 2nd ed. Philadelphia, Pa: WB Saunders; 1998.

Portney LG, Roy SH. Electromyography and nerve conduction velocity tests. In: O'Sullivan SB, Schmitz TJ, eds. *Physical Rehabilitation: Assessment and Treatment.* 4th ed. Philadelphia, Pa: FA Davis; 2001: 213-256.

Schaumberg HH, Berger AR, Thomas PK. *Disorders of Peripheral Nerves.* 2nd ed. Philadelphia, Pa: FA Davis; 1991.

Smorto MP, Basmajian JV. *Electrodiagnosis: A Handbook for Neurologists.* Hagerstown, Md: Harper and Row; 1977.

Spinner M. *Injuries to the Major Branches of Peripheral Nerves of the Forearm.* 2nd ed. Philadelphia, Pa: WB Saunders; 1978.

Sunderland S. *Nerve and Nerve Injuries.* 2nd ed. New York: Churchill Livingstone; 1990.

Sunderland S. *Nerve Injuries and Their Repair: A Critical Appraisal.* New York: Churchill Livingstone; 1991.

Selected Technical Terms

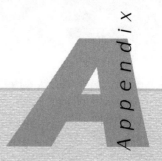

Reprinted with permission from Johnson E, ed. Practical Electromyography. *2nd ed. Baltimore, Md: Williams & Wilkins; 1988.*

amplifier: A device that multiplies its input voltage, current, or power by a fixed or controllable factor, usually without altering its waveform. The output of a voltage or current amplifier may be used as the input to some other low-energy-requiring circuit or indicating device. The output of a power amplifier is typically used to drive loudspeakers, mechanical pen writers, or other energy-transforming devices. An amplifier is sometimes said to be comprised of "stages" that are amplifying circuits arranged in tandem.

amplifier, differential: Used in preamplifiers for EMG, EP, EKG, EEG. It has two recording electrode input terminals (instead of the single input terminal of a conventional amplifier) and a ground or zero-potential terminal. It rejects unwanted potentials originating at a distance and presenting at both input terminals (common mode or in-phase potentials). Potential differences appearing between its two input terminals (differential or out-of-phase potentials) are amplified. Also called balanced amplifier, difference amplifier, long-tailed pair.

artifact: All unwanted potentials which originate outside the tissues being examined. They are also called "noise" when they appear in measurement. An artifact may arise from biological activity, from the electrode or apparatus used in the examination, the power line, or from extrinsic electricity (surrounding the apparatus or patient) (see *noise*).

averager, signal: A signal processing method that aids in the recording of small stimulus evoked potentials which are obscured by noise or artifact. The stimulus is repeated a number of times and the responses are subjected to a special summation technique that causes the random noise portion of the response to become smaller in proportion to the evoked potentials which are coherent in time with each stimulus. This method has also been called noise averaging, response averaging, transient averaging, averaging computer, and ensemble averaging.

common mode rejection: An important property of differential amplifiers that expresses their ability to discriminate against artifact potentials that appear equally at both amplifier input terminals (common mode signals), and to amplify the desired potentials (differential signals) that appear as different signals at the two input terminals. This property may be expressed as the common mode rejection ratio (CMRR) which is the ratio of the amplification for a differential signal to the amplification for a common mode signal applied to the inputs of a differential amplifier.

conduction time indicator: Also termed **time index**. A movable index (or indices) on the trace of the CRT that can be positioned on the recorded waves. The index position is accurately indicated in terms of time, usually in numeric form, measured either from the start of the trace, the shock artifact, or from another index on the screen. Nerve conduction time latencies, action potential durations, or interwave time intervals can thus be conveniently measured without calculations based on sweep times and screen divisions. The term "cursor" is sometimes used.

delay line: A short term electrical dynamic storage device that delays potentials applied to its input so that they appear at its output as if they had occurred (1 to 20 ms) later in time. When an action potential is used to trigger the start of a sweep on the CRT, the delay line permits that portion of the potential immediately preceding the trigger point to be seen on the CRT.

digital system: A system, or circuit, handling or processing information in terms of numbers and utilizing circuits which operate in the manner of switches, having two (on-off) or more discrete positions. The simplest and most common digital system is the binary system. In contrast to analog systems where continuously varying voltages represent the signal being processed, digital systems utilize voltages that jump to various predetermined levels. Patterns of these voltage levels represent, in coded form, the information being processed (see analog-to-digital converter, and digital-to-analog converter).

direct current (DC): A unidirectional current. An intermittent or time-varying current that has a net flow in one direction; is called pulsating DC or DC with an AC component.

filter: In an EMG system, a circuit usually comprised of capacitors and resistors that modifies or adjusts the high and low frequency limit of the amplifier frequency response curve.

frequency: The rate in cycles per second that an AC signal alternates. The unit of frequency is the Hertz (Hz).

frequency response: Describes the speed range (slowest to fastest) of potential waveform changes that will be displayed by the EMG apparatus. Stated as a range (band) of frequencies of sine wave test signals for which the amplification will be uniform. Amplification will decrease progressively for sine wave test signals at frequencies above and below the frequency response band. The frequency between the lower and upper frequency is called bandwidth. The amplifier frequency response bandwidth is often defined by two frequencies, one at the low end, the other at the high end, where amplification falls to 70 percent of its midband value.

ground: The lowest potential terminal in a system. In power distribution systems a terminal that is usually physically connected to a conductor in intimate contact with the earth. Sometimes referred to as the earth terminal. Frame and chassis portions of electrical systems are almost always connected to ground to avoid the possibility of their assuming other random potentials which might be either dangerous or cause electrical interference within the system.

Hertz (Hz): Cycles per second.

impedance: Hindrance to electrical current flow in an AC circuit hence comparable in simplified terms to resistance in DC circuits. Impedance considers the effective capacitance and inductance as well as resistance of AC circuits. A large capacitance has low impedance since it easily passes an AC current. A high resistance has high impedance since it diminishes current flow.

noise: Any potential other than that being measured. Commonly applied to spurious potentials originating within the apparatus or electrodes (see artifact, interference, RMS voltage).

polarity sense, display: Many electrophysiological records are published with an upward deflection denoting a negative potential on the active electrode. Engineering and scientific convention has dictated an upward deflection for a positive potential. When the EMG apparatus utilizes a single multicontact connector for the electrodes (which cannot be reversed) the polarity sense of the equipment is usually fixed and specified. When separate input terminals are provided for each lead wire to the electrodes, the user may determine by selecting the appropriate connections, either positive or negative upward conventions.

preamplifier: The first stage or stages of an EMG amplifier system. It must have a high input impedance, common mode rejection and low noise as well as a large dynamic range. Its performance is important to the quality of the EMG system.

resistance: A property of matter to hinder the flow of direct electric current. Resistance is expressed in ohms and is derived by dividing the voltage impressed by the current that flows. Resistance (R) = Voltage (E) divided by the Current (I).

signal: Any potential, waveform, or intelligence that is communicated, detected, transmitted or processed within a system. It is usually in the form of a voltage or current within the system. Power supplies and other voltages and currents, whose function is to power, excite or drive active elements within the system, are not signals.

stimulator, ground free (isolated): Used in nerve conduction studies to minimize stimulus artifact. A ground free stimulus output circuit has no connection to the common system ground thereby removing a possible path for injection of undesirable artifact via the patient to the EMG amplifier input ground terminal.

storage, display: A means for retaining, usually on the screen of a cathode ray tube, a transient waveform for study or analysis, together with a means for erasing such information to permit the storage of new data.

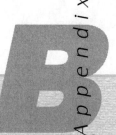

Electromyography and Neuromuscular Definitions

Reprinted from AAEE glossary of terms in clinical electromyography. Muscle & Nerve. 1987;10:G1-G60, with permission of the American Association of Electromyography and Electrodiagnosis ©1987. The Glossary was compiled by the AAEE Nomenclature Committee (C. Jablecki, C. Bolton, W. Bradley, W. Brown, F. Buchthal, R. Cracco, E. Johnson, G. Kraft, E. Lambert, H. Lüders, D. Ma, J. Simpson, and E. Stälberg).

action potential (AP): Strictly defined, the all-or-none, self-propagating, non-decrementing voltage change recorded from an excitable cell. The source of the action potential should be specified, eg, nerve (fiber) action potential or muscle (fiber) action potential. Commonly, the term refers to the nearly synchronous summated action potentials of a group of cells (eg, motor unit potential). To avoid ambiguity in reference to the recording of nearly synchronous summated action potentials of nerve and muscle as done in nerve conduction studies, it is recommended that the terms compound nerve action potential and compound muscle action potential be used.

active electrode: see *recording electrode*.

amplitude: With reference to an action potential, the maximum voltage difference between two points, usually baseline to peak or peak to peak. By convention, the amplitude of the compound muscle action potential is measured from the baseline to the most negative peak. In contrast, the amplitude of a compound sensory nerve action potential, motor unit potential, fibrillation potential, positive sharp wave, fasciculation potential, and most other action potentials is measured from the most positive to the most negative peak.

anode: The positive terminal of a source of electrical current.

antidromic: Said of an action potential or of the stimulation causing the action potential that propagates in the direction opposite to the normal (dromic or orthodromic) one for that fiber (ie, conduction along motor fibers toward the spinal cord and conduction along sensory fibers away from the spinal cord). Contrast with orthodromic.

artifact: A voltage change generated by a biological or nonbiological source other than the ones of interest. The stimulus artifact is the potential recorded at the time the stimulus is applied and includes the electrical or shock artifact, which is a potential due to the volume-conducted electrical stimulus. The stimulus and shock artifacts usually precede the activity of interest. A movement artifact refers to a change in the recorded activity due to movement of the recording electrodes.

baseline: The potential difference recorded from the biological system of interest while the system is at rest.

bipolar needle electrode: A recording electrode with two insulated wires side by side in a metal cannula whose bare tips act as the active and reference electrodes. The metal cannula may be grounded.

bizarre high-frequency discharge: see *complex repetitive discharge*.

cathode: The negative terminal of a source of electrical current.

clinical electromyography: Loosely used to refer to all electrodiagnostic studies of peripheral nerves and muscle (see *electrodiagnosis*).

coaxial needle electrode: see *concentric needle electrode.*

complex action potential: see *serrated action potential.*

complex motor unit potential: see *serrated action potential.*

complex repetitive discharge: Polyphasic or serrated action poten-tials that may begin spontaneously or after a needle movement. They have a uniform frequency, shape, and amplitude, with abrupt onset, cessation, or change in configuration. Amplitude ranges from 100 μV to 1 μV and frequency of discharge from 5 to 100 Hz.

compound action potential: Evoked response from a muscle by a single electrical stimulus to its motor nerve. By convention, the compound action potential elicited by supramaximal stimulation is used for motor nerve conduction studies. The recording electrodes should be placed so that the initial deflection of the evoked potential is negative. The latency, commonly called motor latency, is the latency (ms) to the onset of the first negative phase. The amplitude (mV) is the baseline-to-peak amplitude of the first negative phase, unless otherwise specified. The duration (ms) refers to the duration of the first negative phase, unless otherwise specified. Normally, the configuration of the compound action potential (usually biphasic) is quite stable with repeated stimuli at slow rates (1 to 5 Hz) (see *repetitive stimulation, compound mixed nerve action potential, compound motor nerve action potential, compound nerve action potential, compound sensory nerve action potential,* and *compound muscle action potential*).

compound mixed nerve action potential: A compound nerve action potential is considered to have been evoked from afferent and efferent fibers if the recording electrodes detect activity on a mixed nerve with the electrical stimulus applied to a segment of the nerve that contains both afferent and efferent fibers.

compound motor nerve action potential: A compound nerve action potential is considered to have been evoked from efferent fibers to a muscle if the recording electrodes detect activity only in a motor nerve or a motor branch of a mixed nerve, or if the electrical stimulus is applied only to such a nerve or a ventral root. The amplitude, latency, duration, and phases should be noted (see *compound nerve action potential*)

compound muscle action potential: The summation of nearly synchronous muscle fiber action potentials recorded from a muscle commonly produced by stimulation of the nerve supplying the muscle either directly or indirectly. Baseline-to-peak amplitude, duration, and latency of the negative phase should be noted, along with details of the method of stimulation and recording.

compound nerve action potential: The summation of nearly synchronous nerve fiber action potentials recorded from a nerve trunk, commonly produced by stimulation of the nerve directly or indirectly. Details of the method of stimulation and recording should be specified, together with the fiber type (sensory, motor, or mixed).

compound sensor nerve action potential: A compound nerve action potential is considered to have been evoked from afferent fibers if the recording electrodes detect activity only in a sensory nerve or in a sensory branch of a mixed nerve, or if the electrical stimulus is applied to such a nerve or a dorsal nerve root, or an adequate stimulus is applied synchronously to sensory receptors. The amplitude, latency, duration, and configuration should be noted. Generally, the amplitude is measured as the maximum peak-to-peak voltage, the latency as the peak latency to the negative peak, and the duration as the interval from the first deflection of the waveform from the baseline to its final return to the baseline. The compound sensory nerve action potential has been referred to as the sensory response or sensory potential.

concentric needle electrode: Recording electrode that measures the potential difference between the bare tip of a central insulated wire in the bare shaft of a metal cannula. The bare tip of the central wire (active electrode) is flush with the bevel of the cannula (reference electrode).

conduction block: Failure of an action potential to be conducted past a particular point in the nervous system. In practice, a conduction block is documented by demonstration of a reduction in amplitude of an evoked potential greater than that normally seen with electrical stimulation at two different points on a nerve trunk; anatomical nerve variations and technical factors related to nerve stimulation must be excluded as the source of the reduction in amplitude.

conduction velocity: Speed of propagation of an action potential along a nerve or muscle fiber. The nerve fiber studied (motor, sensory, autonomic, or mixed) should be specified. For a nerve trunk the maximum conduction velocity is calculated from the latency of the evoked potential (muscle or nerve) at maximal or supramaximal intensity of stimulation at two different points. The distance between the two points (conduction distance) is divided by the difference between the corresponding latencies (conduction time). The calculated velocity represents the conduction velocity of the fastest fibers and is expressed as meters per second (m/sec). As commonly used, the term conduction velocity refers to the maximum conduction velocity. By specialized techniques, the conduction velocity of other fibers can be determined as well and should be specified, eg, minimum conduction velocity.

contraction: A voluntary or involuntary reversible muscle shorten-ing that may or may not be accompanied by action potentials from muscle.

cycles per second (C/sec or CPS): Unit of frequency. . Preferred equivalent is Hertz (Hz).

delay: Interval between onset of oscilloscope sweep and onset of a stimulus. Has been used in the past to designate the interval from the stimulus to the response. Compare with latency.

denervation potential: Use of term discouraged (see *fibrillation potential*).

depolarization: A decrease in the electrical potential difference across a membrane from any cause, to any degree, relative to the nominal resting potential.

discharge frequency: The rate of repetition of an action potential. When potentials occur in groups, the rate of recurrence of the group and the rate of repetition of the individual components in the groups should be specified.

discrete activity: The pattern of electrical activity at full voluntary contraction of the muscle is reduced to the extent that each individual motor unit potential can be identified. The firing frequency of each of these potentials should be specified together with the force contraction.

distal latency: see *motor latency* and *sensory latency*.

"Dive Bomber" potential: Use of term discouraged (see preferred term, *myotonic discharge*).

duration: The time during which something exists or acts. The duration of individual potential waveforms is defined as the interval from the first deflection from the baseline to its final return to the baseline, unless otherwise specified. One common exception is the duration of the (compound action potential, which usually refers to the interval from the deflection of the first negative phase from the baseline to its return to the baseline. The duration of a single electrical stimulus refers to the interval of the applied current or voltage. The duration of recurring stimuli or action potentials refers to the interval from the beginning to the end of the series.

earthing electrode: Synonymous with *ground electrode*.

electrical artifact: see *artifact*.

electrical silence: The absence of measurable electrical activity due to biological or nonbiological sources. The sensitivity, or signal-to-noise level, of the recording system should be specified.

electrode: A device capable of conducting electricity. The material (metal, fabric), size, configuration (disc, ring, needle), and location (surface, intramuscular intracranial) should be specified. Electrodes may be used to record an electrical potential difference (recording electrodes) or to apply an electrical current (stimulating electrodes). In both cases, two electrodes are always required. Depending on the relative size and location of the electrodes, however, the stimulating or recording condition may be referred to as "monopolar" (see ground electrode, recording electrode, and stimulating electrode. Also see specific needle electrode configurations: monopolar, concentric, bipolar, and multilead needle electrodes).

electromyelography: The recording and study of electrical activity from the spinal cord. The term is also used to refer to studies of electrical activity from the cauda equina.

electromyograph: An instrument for detecting and displaying ac-tion potentials from muscle and nerve.

electromyography (EMG): Strictly defined, the recording and study of insertional, spontaneous, and voluntary electrical activity of muscle. It is commonly used to refer to nerve conduction studies as well (see *clinical electromyography* and the more general term, *electrophysiologic evaluation*).

electroneurography: The recording and study of the action potentials of peripheral nerves (see preferred term, *nerve conduction studies*, and the more general term, *electrophysiologic evaluation*).

electrophysiologic evaluation: General term used to refer to the recording of responses of nerves and muscle to electrical stimulation and the recording of insertional, spontaneous, and voluntary action potentials from muscle.

end-plate activity: Spontaneous electrical activity recorded with a needle electrode close to muscle endplates. May be either of two forms:

✦   **Monophasic**: Low-amplitude (10 to 20 µV), short-duration (0.5 to 1 msec), monophasic (negative) potentials that occur in a dense, steady pattern and are restricted to a localized area of the muscle. Because of the multitude of different potentials occurring, the exact frequency, although appearing to be high, cannot be defined. These potentials are miniature end-plate potentials recorded extracellularly. This form of end-plate activity has been referred to as end-plate noise and is associated with a sound not unlike that of a seashell, which has been called a seashell noise or roar.

✦   **Biphasic**: Moderate-amplitude (100 to 300 µV), short-duration (2 to 4 msec), biphasic (negative-positive) spike potentials that occur irregularly in short bursts with a high frequency (50 to 100 Hz), restricted to a localized area within the muscle. These potentials are generated by muscle fibers excited by activity in nerve terminals. These potentials have been referred to incorrectly, as "nerve" potentials.

end-plate noise: see *end-plate activity, monophasic.*

end-plate potential: Graded, nonpropagated potential recorded by microelectrodes from muscle fibers in the region of the neuromuscular junction.

evoked action potential: Action potential elicited by a stimulus.

evoked compound muscle action potential: The electrical activity of a muscle produced by stimulation of the nerves supplying the muscle. Baseline-to-peak amplitude of the negative phase duration of the negative phase, and latency should be measured, details of the method of stimulation should be recorded.

evoked potential: Electrical waveform elicited by and temporally related to a stimulus, most commonly an electrical stimulus delivered to a sensory receptor or nerve, or applied directly to a discrete area of the brain, spinal cord, or muscle.

excitability: Capacity to be activated by or react to a stimulus.

fasciculation: The random, spontaneous twitching of a group of muscle fibers which may be visible through the skin. The electrical activity associated with the spontaneous contraction is called the fasciculation potential. Compare with myokymia.

fasciculation potential: The electrical potential associated with fasciculation which has dimension of a motor unit potential that occurs spontaneously as a single discharge. Most commonly these potentials occur sporadically and are termed "single fasciculation potentials." Occasionally, the potentials occur as a grouped discharge and are termed "grouped fasciculation potentials." The occurrence of large numbers of either simple or grouped fasciculations may produce a writhing vermicular movement of the skin called myokymia. Use of the terms benign fasciculation and malignant fasciculation is discouraged. Instead, the configuration of the potentials, peak-to-peak amplitude, duration, number of phases, and stability of configuration, in addition to frequency of occurrence, should be specified.

fatigue: Reduction in the force of contraction of muscle fibers as a result of repeated use or electric stimulation. More generally, it is a state of depressed responsiveness resulting from protracted activity and requiring appreciable recovery time.

fiber density: Anatomically, fiber density is a measure of the number of muscle or nerve fibers per unit area. In single-fiber EMG, the fiber density is the mean number of muscle fiber potentials under voluntary control encountered during a systematic search.

fibrillation potential: The electrical activity associated with fibrillating muscle fibers, reflecting the action potential of a single muscle fiber. The action potentials may occur spontaneously or after movement of the needle electrode. The potentials usually occur repetitively and regularly. Classically, the potentials are biphasic spikes of short duration (usually less than 5 ms) with an initial positive phase and a peak-to-peak amplitude of less than 1 μV. The firing rate has a wide range (1 to 50 Hz) and often decreases just before cessation of an individual discharge. A high-pitched regular sound is associated with the discharge of fibrillation potentials and has been described in the old literature as "rain on a tin roof." In addition to this classic form of fibrillation potentials, positive sharp waves may also be recorded from fibrillating muscle fibers; the difference in the configuration of the potentials is due to the position of the recording electrode.

firing pattern: Qualitative and quantitative description of the sequence of discharge of potential waveforms recorded from muscle or nerve.

firing rate: Frequency of repetition of a potential. The relationship of the frequency to the occurrence of other potentials and the force of muscle contraction may be described (see discharge frequency).

frequency: Number of complete cycles of a repetitive waveform in 1 second. Measured in Hertz (I), a unit preferred to its equivalent, cycles per second (C/sec).

F wave: A late compound action potential evoked intermittently from a muscle by a supramaximal electrical stimulus to the nerve. Compared win the maximal amplitude compound action potential of the same muscle, the F wave has a reduced amplitude and variable configuration and a longer and more variable latency. It can be found in many muscles of the upper and lower extremities, and the latency is longer with more distal sites of stimulation. The F wave is due to antidromic activation of motor neurons. It was named by Magladery and McDougal in 1950.

"giant" motor unit action potential: Use of term discouraged. It refers to a motor unit potential with a peak-to-peak amplitude and duration much greater than the range recorded in corresponding muscles in normal subjects of similar age. Quantitative measurements of amplitude and duration are preferable.

ground electrode: An electrode connected to a large conducting body (such as the earth) used as a common return for an electrical circuit and as an arbitrary zero potential reference point.

grouped discharge: Intermittent repetition of a group of action potentials with the same or nearly the same waveform and a relatively short interpotential interval within the group in comparison with the time interval between each group. It may occur spontaneously or with voluntary activity and may be regular or irregular in its firing pattern.

Hertz (Hz): Unit of frequency representing cycles per second.

Hoffman reflex: see *H Reflex*.

H reflex: A late compound muscle action potential having a consistent latency evoked regularly, when present, from a muscle by an electrical stimulus to the nerve. It is regularly found only in a limited group of physiologic extensors, particularly the calf muscles. The reflex is most easily obtained with the cathode positioned proximal to the anode. Compared with the maximal amplitude compound action potential of the same muscle, the H wave has a reduced amplitude, a longer latency, and a lower optimal stimulus intensity; its configuration is constant. The latency is longer with more distal sites of stimulation. A stimulus intensity sufficient to elicit a maximal-amplitude compound action potential reduces or abolishes the H wave. The H wave is thought to be due to a spinal reflex, the Hoffman reflex, with electrical stimulation of afferent fibers in the mixed nerve to the muscle and activation of motor neurons to the muscle through a monosynaptic connection in the spinal cord. The reflex and wave are named in honor of Hoffman's description (1918). Compare with F Wave.

insertional activity: Electrical activity caused by insertion or movement of a needle electrode. The amount of the activity may be described qualitatively as normal, reduced, increased, or prolonged.

interference pattern: Electrical activity recorded from a muscle with a needle electrode during maximal voluntary effort, in which identification of each of the contributing action potentials is not possible, because of the overlap or interference of one potential with another. When no individual potentials can be identified, this is known as full interference pattern. A reduced interference pattern is one in which some of the individual potentials may be identified while other individual potentials cannot be identified because of overlapping. The term discrete activity is used to describe the electrical activity recorded when each of the motor unit potentials can be identified. It is important that the force of contraction associated with the interference pattern be specified.

involuntary activity: Action potentials that are not under voluntary control. The condition under which they occur should be described (eg, spontaneous, or, if elicited by a stimulus, the nature of the stimulus). Compare with spontaneous activity.

latency: Interval between the onset of stimulus and the onset of a response unless otherwise specified. Latency always refers to the onset unless specified, as in peak latency.

membrane instability: Tendency of a cell membrane to depolarize spontaneously or after mechanical irritation or voluntary activation.

miniature end-plate potential: When recorded with microelectrodes, monophasic negative discharges with amplitudes less than 100 µV and duration of 4 ms or less, occurring irregularly and recorded in an area of muscle corresponding to the myoneural junction. They are thought to be due to small quantities (quanta) of acetylcholine released spontaneously. Compare with end-plate activity.

monopolar needle electrode: A solid wire, usually of stainless steel, coated, except at its tip, with an insulating material. Variations in voltage between the tip of the needle (active or exploring electrode) positioned in a muscle and a conductive plate on the skin surface or a bare needle in subcutaneous tissue (reference electrode) are measured. By convention, this recording condition is referred to as a monopolar needle electrode recording; it should be emphasized, however, that potential differences are always recorded between two electrodes.

motor latency: Interval between the onset of a stimulus and the onset of the resultant compound muscle action potential. The term may be qualified as proximal motor latency or distal motor latency, depending on the relative position of the stimulus.

motor point: The point over a muscle where a contraction of a muscle may be elicited by a minimal intensity, short-duration electrical stimulus.

motor unit: The anatomical unit of an anterior horn cell, its axon, the neuromuscular junctions, and all the muscle fibers innervated by the axon.

motor unit action potential (MUAP): see synonym, motor unit potential.

motor unit potential (MUP): Action potential reflecting the electrical activity of that part of a single anatomical motor unit that is within the recording range of an electrode. The action potential is characterized by its consistent appearance with and relationship to the force of a voluntary contraction of a muscle. The following parameters should be specified, quantitatively if possible, after the recording electrode is placed so as to minimize the rise time (which by convention should be less than 0.5 msec), which generally also maximizes the amplitude:

1. Configuration
   A. Amplitude, peak-to-peak (μV or mV)
   B. Duration, total (ms)
   C. Number of phases (monophasic, biphasic, triphasic, tetraphasic, polyphasic)
   D. Direction of each phase (negative, positive)
   E. Number of turns of serrated potential
   F. Variation of shape with consecutive discharges

2. Recruitment characteristics
   A. Threshold of activation (first recruited, low threshold, high threshold)
   B. Onset frequency (Hz)
   C. Recruitment frequency (Hz) or Recruitment interval (ms) of individual potentials

multilead electrode: Three or more insulated wires inserted through a common metal cannula with their bared tips at an aperture in the cannula and flush with the outer circumference of the cannula. The arrangement of the bare tips relative to the axis of the cannula and the distance between each tip should be specified.

muscle action potential: Strictly defined, the term refers to the action potential recorded from a single muscle fiber. However, the term is commonly used to refer to a compound muscle action potential (see *compound muscle action potential*).

muscle fiber conduction velocity: The speed of propagation of a single muscle fiber action potential, usually expressed as meters per second. The muscle fiber conduction velocity is usually less than most nerve conduction velocities, varies with the rate of discharge of the muscle fiber, and requires special techniques for measurement.

myokymia: Involuntary, continuous quivering muscle fibers which may be visible through the skin as a vermiform movement. It is associated with spontaneous, rhythmic discharge of motor unit potentials.

myokymic discharges: Action potentials with the configuration of motor unit potentials that occur spontaneously, recur regularly, and may be associated with clinical myokymia. Two distinct firing patterns are recognized. Commonly, the discharges are grouped with a short period (up to a few seconds) of firing at a uniform rate (2 to 20 Hz) followed by a short period (up to a few seconds) of silence, with repetition of the same sequence for a particular potential. Less commonly, the potential recurs continuously at a fairly uniform firing rate (1 to 5 Hz). Myokymic discharges are a subclass of grouped discharges and repetitive discharges.

myopathic motor unit potential: It is used to refer to low-amplitude, short-duration, polyphasic motor unit action potentials. The term incorrectly implies specific diagnostic significance of motor unit potential configuration (see motor unit potential).

myopathic recruitment: It is used to describe an increase in the number of and firing rate of motor unit potentials compared with normal for the strength of muscle contraction.

myotonic discharge: Repetitive discharge of 20 to 80 Hz of biphasic (positive-negative) spike potential less than 5 ms in duration or monophasic positive waves of 5 to 20 ms recorded after needle insertion, or less commonly after voluntary muscle contraction or muscle percussion. The amplitude and frequency of the potentials must both wax and wane to be identified as myotonic discharges. This change produces a characteristic musical sound in the audio display of the electromyograph due to the corresponding charge in pitch, which has been likened to the sound of a "dive bomber."

myotonic response: Delayed relaxation of muscle after voluntary contraction or percussion and associated with a myotonic discharge.

needle electrode: An electrode for recording or stimulating, shaped like a needle (see specific electrodes: *bipolar needle electrode, concentric needle electrode, monopolar needle electrode, multilead electrode*).

nerve action potential: Strictly defined, refers to an action potential recorded from a single nerve fiber. The term is commonly used to refer to the compound nerve action potential (see *compound nerve action potential*).

nerve conduction studies: Refers to all aspects of electrophysiologic evaluation of peripheral nerves. However, the term is generally used to refer to the recording and measurement of a compound nerve and compound muscle action potential elicited in response to a single supramaximal electrical stimulus under standardized conditions that permit establishment of normal ranges of amplitude, duration, and latency of evoked potentials and the calculation of the maximum conduction velocity of individual nerves (see compound nerve action potential, compound muscle action potential, conduction velocity, and repetitive stimulation).

nerve conduction (NCV): Loosely used to refer to the maximum nerve conduction velocity (see *conduction velocity*).

nerve potential: Equivalent to nerve action potential. Also commonly, but inaccurately, used to refer to the biphasic form of end-plate activity. The latter use is incorrect because muscle fibers, not nerve fibers, are the source of these potentials.

neuropathic motor unit potential: It is used to refer to abnormally high-amplitude, long-duration, polyphasic motor unit potentials. The term incorrectly implies a specific diagnostic significance of a motor unit potential configuration.

neuropathic recruitment: It has been used to describe a recruitment pattern with decreased number of motor unit potentials firing at a rapid rate (see preferred terms, *discrete activity, reduced interference pattern*).

noise: Strictly defined, an artifact consisting of low-amplitude, random potentials produced by an amplifier and unrelated to the input signal. It is most apparent when high gains are used. It is loosely used to refer to end-plate noise. Compare with end-plate activity.

orthodromic: Said of action potentials or stimuli eliciting action potentials propagated in the same direction as physiological conduction (eg, motor nerve conduction away from the spinal cord and sensory nerve conduction toward the spinal cord). Contrast with antidromic.

peak latency: Interval between the onset of a stimulus and a specified peak of the evoked potential (usually the negative peak).

phase: That portion of a wave between the departure from and the return to the baseline.

polarization: As used in neurophysiology, the presence of an electrical potential difference across an excitable cell membrane. The potential across the membrane of a cell when it is not excited by input or spontaneously active is termed the Resting Potential; it is at a steady state with regard to the electrical potential difference across the membrane. Depolarization describes a decrease in polarization to any degree, relative to the normal resting potential. Hyperpolarization describes an increase in polarization relative to the resting potential. Repolarization describes an increase in polarization from the depolarized state toward, but not above, the normal or resting potential.

positive sharp wave: Strictly defined, one form of electrical activity associated with fibrillating muscle fibers. It is recorded as a biphasic, positive-negative action potential initiated by needle movement and recurring in a uniform, regular pattern at a rate of 2 to 50 Hz, which may decrease just before cessation of discharge. The amplitude and duration vary considerably but the initial positive deflection is usually less than 5 ms in duration and up to 1 mV in amplitude. The negative phase is of low amplitude, with a duration of 10 to 100 ms. A sequence of positive sharp waves is commonly referred to as a train of positive sharp waves. Positive sharp waves are recorded from the damaged area of fibrillating muscle fibers. Loosely defined, positive sharp waves refer to any action potential recorded with the waveform of a positive wave, without reference to the firing pattern or method of generation.

pseudomyotonic discharge: Use of term discouraged. It has been used to refer to different phenomena, including (1) myotonic discharges occurring in the presence of a neurogenic disease (2) complex repetitive discharges, and (3) repetitive discharges that wax or wane in either frequency or amplitude but not in both.

recording electrode: Device used to monitor electrical current or potential. All electrical recordings require two electrodes. The electrode close to the source of the activity to be recorded is called the active electrode, and the other electrode is called the reference electrode. Active electrode is synonymous with the older terminology G1 or Grid 1, and the reference electrode with G2 or Grid 2. By current convention, a potential difference that is negative at the active electrode relative to the reference electrode causes an upward deflection on the oscilloscope screen. The term "monopolar recording" is not recommended, because all recording requires two electrodes; however, it is commonly used to describe the use of an intramuscular needle exploring electrode in combination with a surface disc or subcutaneous needle reference electrode.

recruitment: The orderly activation of the same and new motor units with increasing strength of voluntary muscle contraction (see *motor unit potential*).

recruitment frequency: Firing rate of a motor unit potential when an additional motor unit potential first appears during gradually increasing strength of voluntary muscle contraction.

recruitment interval: The interdischarge interval between two consecutive discharges of a motor unit potential when an additional motor unit potential first appears during gradually increasing strength of voluntary muscle contraction. The reciprocal of the recruitment interval is the recruitment frequency.

recruitment pattern: A qualitative and/or quantitative description of the sequence of appearance of motor unit potentials with increasing strength of voluntary muscle contraction. The recruitment frequency and recruitment interval are two quantitative measures commonly used (see *interference pattern* for qualitative terms commonly used).

repetitive discharges: General term for the recurrence of an action potential with the same or nearly the same form. The term may refer to recurring potentials recorded in muscle at rest, during voluntary contraction, or in response to single nerve stimulus. The discharge may be named for the number of times a potential recurs in a group (eg, double discharge, triple discharge, multiple discharge, coupled discharge) or other characteristics (eg, complex repetitive discharge, myokymic discharge).

repetitive stimulation: The technique of utilizing repeated supramaximal stimulation of a nerve while quantitatively recording compound action potentials from muscles innervated by the nerve. It should be described in terms of the frequency of stimuli and number of stimuli (or duration of the total group).

residual latency: Refers to the calculated time difference between the measured distal latency of a motor nerve and the expected distal latency, calculated by dividing the distance between the stimulus cathode and the active recording electrode by the maximum conduction velocity measured in a more proximal segment of a nerve.

rise time: By convention, the shortest interval from the nadir of a positive phase to the peak of negative phase of a compound action potential.

sensory peak latency: Interval between the onset of a stimulus and the peak of the negative phase of the compound sensory nerve action potential. Note that the term "latency" refers to the interval between the onset of a stimulus and the onset of a response.

serrated action potential: An action potential waveform with several changes in direction (turns) which do not cross the baseline. This term is preferred to the term complex action potential (see *turns*).

single fiber needle electrode: A needle electrode with a small recording surface (usually 25 microns in diameter) permitting the recording of single muscle fiber action potentials (see single fiber electromyography).

somatosensory evoked potential (SSEP): Electrical waves recorded from the head or trunk in response to electrical or physiological stimulation of peripheral sensory fibers. Recordings over the spine may be referred to as spinal evoked potentials.

spinal evoked potential: Electrical wave recorded over the spine in response to electrical stimulation of peripheral sensory fibers (see *somatosensory evoked potential*).

spontaneous activity: Action potentials recorded from muscle or nerve at rest after insertional activity has subsided and when there is no voluntary contraction or external stimulus. Compare with involuntary activity.

stimulating electrode: Device used to apply electrical current. All electrical stimulation requires two electrodes; the negative terminal is termed the cathode and the positive terminal, the anode. By convention, the stimulating electrodes are called "bipolar" if they are roughly equal in size and separated by less than 5 cm. The stimulating electrodes are called "monopolar" if the cathode is smaller in size than the anode and is separated from the anode by more than 5 cm. Electrical stimulation for nerve conduction studies generally requires application of the cathode to produce depolarization of the nerve trunk fibers. If the anode is inadvertently placed between the cathode and the recording electrodes, a focal block of nerve conduction (Anodal Block) may occur and cause a technically unsatisfactory study.

stimulus: Any external agent, state, or change that is capable of influencing the activity of a cell, tissue, or organism. In clinical nerve conduction studies, an electrical stimulus is generally applied to a nerve or a muscle. The electrical stimulus may be described in absolute terms or with respect to the evoked potential of the nerve or muscle. In absolute terms, the electrical stimulus has a strength or intensity measured in voltages (volts) or current (milliamperes) and a duration (milliseconds). With respect to the evoked potential, the stimulus may be graded as subthreshold, threshold, submaximal, maximal, or supramaximal. A threshold stimulus is that electrical stimulus just sufficient to produce a detectable response. Stimuli less than the threshold stimulus are termed subthreshold the maximal stimulus is the stimulus intensity after which a further increase in the stimulus intensity causes no increase in the amplitude of the evoked potential. Stimuli of intensity below this and above threshold are submaximal. Stimuli of intensity greater than the maximal stimulus are termed supramaximal. Ordinarily, supramaximal stimuli are used for nerve conduction studies. By convention, an electrical stimulus of approximately 20% greater voltage than required for the maximal stimulus may be used for supramaximal stimulation. The frequency, number, and duration of a series of stimuli should be specified.

strength-duration curve: Graphic presentation of the relationship between the intensity (Y axis) and various durations (X axis) of the threshold electrical stimulus for a muscle with the stimulating cathode positioned over the motor point.

temporal dispersion: Relative desynchronization of components of a compound action potential due to different rates of conduction of each synchronously evoked component from the stimulation point to the recording electrode.

terminal latency: Synonymous with preferred term, distal latency (see motor latency and sensory latency).

threshold: The level at which a clear and abrupt transition occurs from one state to another. The term is generally used to refer to the voltage level at which an action potential is initiated in a single axon or a group of axons. It is also operationally defined as the intensity that produced a response in about 50% of equivalent trials.

turns: Changes in direction of a waveform which do not necessarily pass through the baseline. The minimal excursion required to constitute a turn should be specified.

unipolar needle electrode: see *monopolar needle electrode*.

visual evoked potential: Electrical waveforms of biological origin recorded over the cerebrum and elicited by light stimuli.

volume conduction: Spread of current from a potential source through a conducting medium, such as the body tissues.

voluntary activity: In electromyography, the electrical activity recorded from a muscle with consciously controlled muscle contraction. The effort made to contract the muscle (eg, minimal, moderate, or maximal), and the strength of contraction in absolute terms or relative to a maximal voluntary contraction of a normal corresponding muscle should be specified.

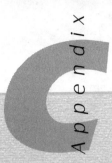

Universal Precautions

Reprinted with permission from Hopp JW, Rogers EA. Aids and the Allied Health Professions. Philadelphia, Pa: FA Davis; 1989.

Universal precautions supplement, but do not replace, responsible practice. In addition, universal precautions propose:

1. Protective barrier use. Gloves should always be used to protect hands from contamination by blood, bloody fluids, and other infectious fluids. Mask and eyewear (or face shields) should be used to protect mucous membranes from droplets or other splatter. Gowns should be worn to protect from spill and splash.

2. Hands, skin, and mucous membranes should be washed immediately and thoroughly if contaminated with blood, bloody fluids, or other infectious fluids.

3. All health care workers should be careful to prevent injuries with needles and other sharp objects. Needles should not be recapped or manipulated by hand in any way. They should be placed in puncture-resistant containers for disposal.

4. Ventilation devices should be readily available for use during resuscitation. Although there is no evidence suggesting that saliva transmits human immunodeficiency virus (HIV), mouth-to-mouth resuscitation should be avoided.

5. Health care workers with open, weeping skin lesions should not give direct patient care or handle patient-care equipment until the lesions heal.

6. Because blood-borne organisms, especially the HIV and cytomegalovirus (CMV), present special risks to fetuses, pregnant employees should be especially careful to follow universal precautions.

Both latex and vinyl gloves, when intact, are barriers to HIV and other blood-borne infectious agents. The type of glove to be used depends on the task of be perform. Use sterile gloves when sterility is needed. Examination gloves (non-sterile latex or vinyl gloves) should be used to protect hands from blood or bloody fluids and from major contamination. Use household rubber gloves (utility gloves) when doing housekeeping tasks involving contact with blood, blood spills, or gross contamination, or when exposed to sharp penetrating objects such as those used in autopsies or associated with auto accidents.

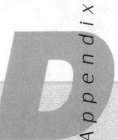

Suggested Format for Reporting Electromyography Nerve Conduction Studies Consultation

Referring diagnosis:
Testing requested:
Referred by:
Date:
Problem:
Subjective (Hx):

Objective (brief clinical exam):
   Observation:
   Palpation:
   ROM:
   Neuro:
   Sensation:
   MMT:
   Reflexes:
   Special Tests:
   Other:

NCV findings summarized (Data Sheet 1):

EMG findings in logical order, muscles tested by peripheral nerve, nerve root distribution, etc. (Data Sheet 2):

Muscle—Comment on spontaneous activity, potentials seen on volition, recruitment of motor units, interference pattern:

Assessment:

Patient's name (any identifying number system also):
Electromyographer's signature:

Report on Electromyographic/ Nerve Conduction Studies Data Sheet

Date:

MEDIAN NERVE

	Latency (msec)		Distance (cm)		Amplitude (mV)		NCV (m/sec)	
Anatomic Site	L	R	L	R	L	R	L	R
Wrist								
Elbow								
Upper arm								
Sensory II								
Sensory III								

ULNAR NERVE

	Latency (msec)		Distance (cm)		Amplitude (mV)		NCV (m/sec)	
Anatomic Site	L	R	L	R	L	R	L	R
Wrist								
Below elbow								
Above elbow								
Upper arm								
Sensory V								
First dorsal Int.								

Patient's Identification

Data Sheet 1. Report on electromyographic/nerve conduction studies.

EMG Report Data Sheet

Date: Patient's Name:

Side	Musc	Nerve Root	Insertional Noise	Fibs	Psw	Fasc	Polys	NMU	Amp	Recruit	Int. pattern/ comments
1											
2											
3											
4											
5											
6											
7											
8											
9											
10											
11											
12											
13											
14											
15											
16											
17											
18											

Data Sheet 2. EMG report.

Index

Build Your Library

Along with this title, we publish numerous products on a variety of topics. We are sure that you will find the below titles to be an essential addition to your library. Order your copies today or contact us for a copy of our latest catalog for additional product information.

INTRODUCTION TO ELECTROMYOGRAPHY AND NERVE CONDUCTION TESTING, SECOND EDITION

John L. Echternach, EdD, PT, ECS, FAPTA
208 pp., Soft Cover (Layflat), 2002,
ISBN 1-55642-529-5, Order #45295, **$28.95**

This text has been completely revised and updated to include the latest information in the area of nerve conduction testing and electromyography. The combination of insightful text, excellent illustrations, and laboratory exercises enable the reader to gain a comprehensive understanding of the topic and develop essential skills for this form of testing.

SPECIAL TESTS FOR ORTHOPEDIC EXAMINATION, SECOND EDITION

Jeff G. Konin, Med, ATC, MPT; Denise L. Wiksten, PhD, ATC; Jerome A. Isear, Jr., MS, PT, ATC; and Holly Brader, MPH, ATC, CHES
352 pp., Soft Cover (Wire-O), 2002,
ISBN 1-55642-591-0, Order #45910, **$33.95**

This text takes a simplistic approach to visualizing and explaining over 150 commonly used orthopedic special tests. Readers benefit from the user-friendly format, as clear and concise text is coupled with excellent photographs to illustrate the subject and clinician positioning. The tests are organized by regions of the body so the reader can easily reference a particular test.

ORTHOTICS: A COMPREHENSIVE CLINICAL APPROACH

Joan Edelstein, MA, PT, FISPO and Jan Bruckner, PhD, PT
192 pp., Hard Cover, 2002, ISBN 1-55642-416-7, Order #44167, **$38.95**

Orthotics: A Comprehensive Clinical Approach is an innovative and comprehensive text that provides essential information about contemporary orthoses to guide the student and clinician in prescribing and utilizing these appliances in neuromuscular, musculoskeletal, and integumentary rehabilitation. Each chapter has interesting "thought" questions and case studies to promote clinical reasoning and problem-solving skills.

Contact Us

SLACK Incorporated, Professional Book Division
6900 Grove Road, Thorofare, NJ 08086
1-800-257-8290/1-856-848-1000, Fax: 1-856-853-5991
orders@slackinc.com or www.slackbooks.com

- -

ORDER FORM

QUANTITY	TITLE	ORDER #	PRICE
	Intro to EMG and Nerve Conduction Testing, Second Edition	45295	**$28.95**
	Special Tests for Orthopedic Examination, Second Edition	45910	**$33.95**
	Orthotics: A Comprehensive Clinical Approach	44167	**$38.95**

Name: _____

Address: _____

City: _____ State: _____ Zip: _____

Phone: _____ Fax: _____

Email: _____

Subtotal	$
Applicable state and local tax will be added to your purchase	$
Handling	$4.50
Total	$

- Check enclosed (Payable to SLACK Incorporated): _____
- Charge my: ___ [AMERICAN EXPRESS] ___ [VISA] ___ [MasterCard]

Account #: _____

Exp. date: _____ Signature: _____

NOTE: *Prices are subject to change without notice. Shipping charges will apply. Shipping and handling charges are non-returnable.*

CODE: 328